W0227693

ACUTE VIRUS INFECTIONS OF POULTRY

CURRENT TOPICS IN VETERINARY MEDICINE AND ANIMAL SCIENCE

ACUTE VIRUS INFECTIONS OF POULTRY

A Seminar in the CEC Agricultural Research Programme, held in Brussels, June 13–14, 1985

Sponsored by the Commission of the European Communities, Directorate-General for Agriculture, Co-ordination of Agricultural Research

Edited by

J.B. McFerran and M.S. McNulty
Veterinary Research Laboratories, Belfast, Northern Ireland

1986 **MARTINUS NIJHOFF PUBLISHERS**
a member of the KLUWER ACADEMIC PUBLISHERS GROUP
DORDRECHT / BOSTON / LANCASTER
for
THE COMMISSION OF THE EUROPEAN COMMUNITIES

Distributors

for the United States and Canada: Kluwer Academic Publishers, 190 Old Derby Street, Hingham, MA 02043, USA
for the UK and Ireland: Kluwer Academic Publishers, MTP Press Limited, Falcon House, Queen Square, Lancaster LA1 1RN, UK
for all other countries: Kluwer Academic Publishers Group, Distribution Center, P.O. Box 322, 3300 AH Dordrecht, The Netherlands

Library of Congress Cataloging-in-Publication Data

Acute virus infections of poultry.

   (Developments in veterinary medicine and animal science)
   1. Virus diseases in poultry--Congresses.
I. McFerran, J. B. II. McNulty, M. S. III. Commission of the European Communities. Coordination of Agricultural Reaearch. IV. Series.
SF995.6.V55A28 1986   636.5'0896925   86-8327
ISBN-13: 978-94-010-8405-5

ISBN-13: 978-94-010-8405-5   e-ISBN-13: 978-94-009-4287-5
DOI: 10.1007/978-94-009-4287-5
EUR 10052 EN

Book information

Publication arranged by: Commission of the European Communities, Directorate-General Information Market and Innovation, Luxembourg

Copyright/legal notice

CONTENTS

PREFACE

This book is based on the proceedings of a seminar on acute viral infections of poultry, which was held in Brussels on 13-14 June 1985. The
aim of the seminar, which was sponsored by the CEC, was to gather information on those infections of immediate or increasing importance. It is
hoped that dissemination of this information will make it easier to har-
monize diagnostic and control measures throughout the member states of the
EEC.

Several points emerge from recent outbreaks of highly pathogenic
avian influenza. In view of the apparent change in pathogenicity of the
virus involved in the outbreak in the USA, infections of domestic poultry,
particularly with H5 and H7 sub-types, should be regarded as a potential
threat, even if the viruses involved are of low pathogenicity. The reasons
for the amount of lateral spread which occurred in the USA outbreak are
still not clear, and it can not be assumed that future outbreaks of highly
pathogenic avian influenza will tend to be self-limiting, as in the past.
The importance of denying access of wild birds, particularly water fowl,
to domestic poultry needs to be re-emphasised. Lastly, there appears to
be increasing support for a combination of slaughter and ring vaccination
to control future outbreaks of spreading avian influenza.

Although pigeon paramyxovirus type 1 can be distinguished from classical strains of Newcastle disease virus, this virus can cause disease in
domestic poultry, as exemplified by the 22 outbreaks in Great Britain in
1984. Feed contaminated with infected pigeon droppings and indeed dead
pigeons was the major factor in the epidemiology of the British outbreaks.
The use of aqueous adjuvanted inactivated vaccines to control the disease
in pigeons appears promising, but none of the available vaccines prevent
either infection of pigeons with the virus or subsequent virus excretion.
There is growing awareness of the presence of other avian paramyxovirus infections in domestic poultry. It is possible that some of these may cause
problems in the future.

While infectious bronchitis is controlled by Mass-type vaccines in
some countries of the EEC, there is evidence in other countries of problems caused by antigenically distinct variant strains. Available evidence

suggests that oil adjuvanted infectious bronchitis vaccines give a better immunity in laying birds than the traditional live vaccines. However, best results with both Mass and variant strain oil adjuvanted vaccines are obtained following priming with live vaccines.

The runting-stunting or malabsorption syndrome is a new disease, principally of broiler chickens, which appeared worldwide in the late 1970s. One of its interesting features is the difference seen in the clinical signs and pathological lesions throughout the EEC. The aetiology is still unknown. Some success in experimentally reproducing the condition in Europe using enterovirvuses and parvoviruses has been reported. Some workers favour a mixed aetiology of viruses and bacteria. Reovirus is considered to have an aetiological role by many North American workers, but there is little evidence for this in Europe.

The chick anaemia agent has many of the physical properties of a parvovirus, but its identity as a virus remains to be confirmed. Available evidence indicates that both parvoviruses and enteroviruses can be egg-transmitted in chickens. As these viruses have been recognised in chickens only very recently and are not detected by conventional cell culture techniques, there is a good possibility that they are present in many specific pathogen-free flocks. This, in turn, raises the possibility that virus stocks, including vaccines, grown on tissues derived from infected flocks, may be contaminated with these viruses.

Domestic ducks and geese are growing in economic importance. Work described in this book discusses the relationship of duck fatty kidney syndrome and focal pancreatic necrosis with duck viral hepatitis type 1 and presents evidence that duck viral hepatitis type 2 virus is an astrovirus.

J.B. McFERRAN

M.S. McNULTY

LIST OF PARTICIPANTS

BELGIUM

Dr. J. KISARY
Universite Libre de Bruxelles
Laboratoire de Biophysique et
 Radiobioligie
Rue des Chevaux 67
1640 Rhode - Saint Genese
Bruxelles.

Dr. G. MEULEMANS
National Institute for Veterinary
 Research
99 Groeselenberg
B-1180 Bruxelles.

Professor H. VINDEVOGEL
Clinic of Avian Diseases
Faculty of Veterinary Medicine
University of Liège
45 Rue des Vétérinaires
B-1070 Bruxelles.

FEDERAL REPUBLIC OF GERMANY

Professor E. F. KALETA
Institut fur Geflugelkrankheiten
Justus - Leibig - Universitat
Frankfurter Str 87
D-6300 Giessen.

Professor V. VON BULOW
Institute of Poultry Diseases
Free University of Berlin
Koserstrasse 21
D-1000 Berlin 33 (West).

FRANCE

Dr. G. BENNEJEAN
Laboratoire National de Pathologie
 Aviaire
Les Croix
B.P.9
22440 Ploufragan.

Dr. F. COUDERT
INRA Station de Pathologie Aviaire
 et de Parasitologie
37380 Monnaie.

Dr. D. GAUDRY
Rhône Mérieux
254 Rue Marcel Mérieux
69002 Lyon.

Dr. M. GUITTET
Laboratoire National de Pathologie
 Aviaire
Les Croix
B.P.9
22440 Ploufragan.

Dr. F. LEGROS

Laboratoire National de Pathologie
  Aviaire
Les Croix
B.P.9
22440 Ploufragan.

Dr. J. P. PICAULT

Laboratoire National de Pathologie
  Aviaire
Les Croix
B.P.9
22440 Ploufragan.

GREECE
Dr. G. VEIMOS

Ministry of Agriculture
Directorate of Veterinary Research
Acharnon Str. No. 2
10176 Athens.

ITALY
Dr. P. N. D'APRILE

Istituto Zooprofilattico
  Sperimentale della Venezie
Via G Orus 2
35129 Padova.

Dr. V. PAPPARELLA

Facolta Veterinaire
Via F Delpino
1-80137 Naples.

Professor M. PETEK

Istituto Zooprofilattico
  Sperimentale della Venezie
Via G Orus 2
35129 Padova.

Dr. G. DI MODUGNO

Facolta Veterinaire
Vialle de Caduti di Tutte le Gurre 1
Bari.

THE NETHERLANDS
Dr. F. DAVELAAR

Stichting Gezondheidsdienst Voor
  Pluimvee
Oude Rijksstraatweg 43
Postbus 43
3940 AA Doorn.

Dr. G. KOCH

Central Veterinary Institute
Department of Virology
PO Box 65
8200 AJ Lelystad.

Dr. B. KOUWENHOVEN

Stichting Gezondheidsdienst Voor
  Pluimvee
Oud Rijksstraatweg 43
Postbus 43
3940 AA Doorn.

REPUBLIC OF IRELAND

Dr. R.A.P. CRINION

Faculty of Veterinary Medicine
National University of Ireland
Pembroke Road
Ballsbridge
Dublin 4.

Dr. T. MURPHY

Department of Agriculture
Veterinary Research Laboratory
Abbotstown
Castleknock
Dublin 15.

UNITED KINGDOM

Dr. D. J. ALEXANDER

Poultry Department
Central Veterinary Laboratory
New Haw
Weybridge
Surrey KT15 3NB.

Dr. H. FARMER

Houghton Poultry Research Station
Huntingdon
Cambridgeshire PE17 2DA.

Dr. R.E. GOUGH

Poultry Department
Central Veterinary Laboratory
New Haw
Weybridge
Surrey KT15 3NB.

Dr. R.C. JONES

Sub-department of Avian Medicine
University of Liverpool
Leahurst
Neston
Wirral L64 7TE.

Dr. J. B. McFERRAN

Veterinary Research Laboratories
Stormont
Belfast BT4 3SD.

Dr. M.S. McNULTY

Veterinary Research Laboratories
Stormont
Belfast BT4 3SD.

Dr. J.M. WOOD

Division of Viral Products
National Institute for Biological
 Standards and Control
Holly Hill
Hampstead
London NW3 6RB.

XII

<u>CEC</u>

Mr. J. CONNELL   Commission of the European
                                    Communities
                                  200 Rue de la Loi
                                  1049 Brussels
                                  Belgium.

A LETHAL OUTBREAK OF H5N2 INFLUENZA IN POULTRY IN THE USA:

VIRUS CHARACTERIZATION AND HOST RANGE

J.M. Wood[a], R.G. Webster[b], Y. Kawaoka[b], W.J. Bean[b] and V.F. Nettles[c].

[a]. Division of Viral Products, National Institute for Biological Standards and Control, Holly Hill, Hampstead, London NW3 6 RB, UK
[b]. Department of Virology and Molecular Biology, St Jude Children's Research Hospital, 332 North Lauderdale, P O Box 318, Memphis, Tennessee 38101, U.S.A.
[c]. Southeastern Cooperative Wildlife Disease Study, Department of Parasitology, College of Veterinary Medicine, The University of Georgia, Athens, Georgia 30602, U.S.A.

ABSTRACT

In April 1983, an influenza virus of low virulence appeared in chickens in Pennsylvania, USA. Subsequently, in October 1983, the virus became virulent and caused high mortality in poultry. The causative agent has been identified as an influenza virus of the H5N2 serotype. The haemagglutinin is antigenically closely related to A/Tern/ South Africa/61 (H5N3) and the neuraminidase is similar to that from human H2N2 strains (e.g., A/Japan/305/57) and from some avian influenza virus strains (e.g. A/turkey/Mass/66 [H6N2]).
Experimental infection with the highly pathogenic A/chick/Penn/1370/83 virus produced only mild transient ill-ness in experimentally infected pheasants, little or no clinical signs in ring-billed gulls and pigs, and no clinical signs in pekin ducks. Virus did not replicate efficiently in gulls, ducks and pigs, whereas pheasants shed virus in faeces ($10^{4.7}$ EID_{50}) for at least 15 days. These studies reinforce wildlife surveillance findings indicating that gulls and ducks are unlikely to have transmitted virus between chicken farms during the 1983 outbreak. Although experimental data suggest that wild gallinaceous birds such as pheasants are potentially capable of virus transmission, there has been no evidence of this from wildlife surveil-lance in Pennsylvania.
Experimental infection of chickens with an H5N2 virus isolated from wild ducks one year before the Pennsylvania outbreak or a gull virus (H5N1) isolated in the quarantine area in 1983 resulted in asymptomatic infections and virus replication occurring only in the upper respiratory tract. These studies suggest that if the first H5N2 virus infecting chickens in Pennsylvania originated from waterbirds, changes in host specificity and pathogenicity for chickens and other gallinaceous birds probably occurred during emergence of the Chicken/Penn/83 virus.

INTRODUCTION

Outbreaks of influenza in poultry occur periodically but in most cases these outbreaks involve turkeys and not chickens despite chicken populations often being far greater than the turkey population (Lang, 1982). Highly pathogenic outbreaks caused by H7N7 virus have occurred in chickens in the USA in 1924-25 and in 1929 (Beaudette et al., 1929) and in the USSR, considerable problems have been caused by influenza infections of domestic chickens since 1967 (Alexander, 1982).

Recently, in April 1983, an H5N2 virus was isolated from chickens in Lancaster County, Pennsylvania, USA. The virus caused low mortality (approximately 5%) at first but by October 1983 highly pathogenic H5N2 viruses were isolated from chickens. The birds showed clinical signs after 48 to 96 hours and mortality was as high as 80% after 5 days. The virus spread to Virginia, New Jersey and Maryland and was not limited to chickens; domestic turkeys and gamebirds also were susceptible. By November 1983 a State, Federal and Industry Influenza Task Force was established in an attempt to control the outbreak by combined quarantine restrictions and depopulation of infected flocks. These measures were successful in containing the disease and rapidly reduced the number of infected farms so that by spring 1984 the outbreak had ended. The disease and control procedures led to destruction of over 15 million birds at a cost exceeding $50 million.

A major epidemiological question as the outbreak progressed, was the role of wildlife in the origin and spread of H5N2 virus. The Task Force carried out extensive surveillance on wild life and the results of this survey carried out by Nettles et al. (1985) are presented below. The survey raised several questions about the involvement of certain animal species in the outbreak. We have investigated the susceptibility of gulls, ducks, pheasants and pigs to experimental infection with virulent H5N2 virus and also examined the susceptibility of chickens to infection with H5N2 viruses circulating in wild ducks.

MATERIALS AND METHODS

Viruses

The following H5N2 virus isolates from chickens in Pennsylvania were used in this study: A/chicken/Pennsylvania/1/83, virus isolated from the index case in April 1983 which caused 2.6% mortality and 31% drop in egg production and was designated UP8125 by the National Veterinary Services Laboratory (NVSL), Ames, Iowa) and A/chicken/Pennsylvania/1370/83 virus which was isolated in October 1983 caused up to 80% mortality in chickens and 100% mortality in chicken embryos. These viruses were provided by Dr James Pearson, NVSL. In addition, influenza virus A/swine/Pennsylvania/4/83 (H5N2) was isolated in November 1983 from an asymptomatic infection of a 4-month old pig closely associated with infected chickens and A/duck/NY/189/82 (H5N2) was isolated from a wild mallard in New York in 1982 and was obtained from the influenza virus collection of St Jude Children's Research Hospital (SJCRH). All viruses were grown in 11-day-old embryonated chicken eggs and were studied in a containment laboratory (P3) at SJCRH that had been approved by the US Dept of Agriculture.

Surveillance of wild and domestic animals and man

Surveillance of domestic animals included pigs and free ranging domestic birds associated with poultry farms. Surveillance of wildlife included a) free flying ducks and geese, b) other wild birds associated with poultry farms, poultry manure or poultry carcasses, c) mice and rats associated with poultry houses, d) wild birds reported sick or dead within the quarantine zone. The 4,417 animals tested within the quarantine zone included: 29 black ducks (Anas rubripes); 4 buffleheads (Bucephala albeola); 3 common mergansers (Mergus merganser); 4 common goldeneyes (Bucephala clangula); 14 green-winged teal (Anas crecca); 2 lesser scaup (Aythya affinis); 473 mallards (Anas platyrhynchos); 10 pintails (Anas acuta); 1 ring-necked duck (Aythya collaris); 1 ruddy duck (Oxyura jamaicensis); 1

shoveler (<u>Anas clypeata</u>); 1 wood duck (<u>Aix sponsa</u>); 207 domestic ducks and domestic/wild duck hybrids; 512 Canada geese (<u>Branta canadensis</u>); 16 domestic geese; 13 tundra swans (<u>Cygnus columbianus</u>); 18 herring gulls (<u>Larus argentatus</u>); 189 ring-billed gulls (<u>Larus delawarensis</u>); 85 pen-reared bobwhite quail (<u>Colinus virginianus</u>); 75 pen-reared chuckars (<u>Alectoris chukar</u>); 84 wild ring-necked pheasants (<u>Phasianus colchicus</u>); 178 pen-reared pheasants; 7 domesticated wild turkeys (<u>Meleagris gallopavo</u>); 72 brown-headed cowbirds (<u>Molothrus ater</u>); 201 crows (<u>Corvus brachyrhynchos</u>); 548 house sparrows (<u>Passer domesticus</u>); 14 red-winged blackbirds (<u>Agelaius phoeniceus</u>); 569 starlings (<u>Sturnus vulgaris</u>); 13 miscellaneous passerform birds; 7 mourning doves (<u>Zenaida macroura</u>); 473 pigeons (<u>Columbia livia</u>); 22 black vultures (<u>Coragyps atratus</u>); 8 turkey vultures (<u>Carthartes aura</u>); 9 miscellaneous hawks and owls; 245 house mice (<u>Mus musculus</u>); 24 Norway rats (<u>Rattus norvegicus</u>) and 283 domestic pigs.

Samples taken for virus isolation included tracheal and cloacal swabs of birds, nasal swabs of pigs and man, toes from birds and rodents and lungs from rodents. Swabs and toes were transported to St. Jude Children's Research Hospital in Memphis, Tennessee in 1 ml of phosphate buffered saline (PBS pH7.2) with 50% glycerol and the following antibiotics, 100 units/ml polymyxin B, 250 μg/ml strepto-mycin, 1000 units/ml penicillin, 250 μg/ml gentamicin and 50 units/ml mycostatin. Lung tissue was homogenized with PBS containing antibiotics. All haemagglutinating agents were identified in haemagglutination-inhibition (HI) and neuraminidase-inhibition (NI) tests with specific antisera to the isolated surface antigens of reference influenza viruses or specific antisera to reference paramyxoviruses (Hinshaw et al., 1978). HI tests were performed with receptor-destroying enzyme (RDE)-treated sera (Palmer et al., 1975) and NI tests were done as described previously (WHO, 1973).

Experimental infection of animals

The animals used were 5 to 6-week-old white leghorn chickens, 6-month-old pekin ducks; adult pen-reared ring-necked pheasants, adult and juvenile wild ring-billed gulls and 6-week-old pigs. Gulls were captured by rocket net in Ohio with the assistance of the U.S. Fish and Wildlife Service. All animals were housed in a P3 containment facility in air-filtered compartments.

Inoculation of animals. Birds were exposed to influenza virus by a variety of routes: intravenous, nasal cleft, trachea and oesophagus, and instillation of drops into the eye. Pigs were exposed to virus by the intranasal route.

Specific antibodies

Antisera specific for the isolated haemagglutinin and neuraminidase antigens of the reference strains of influenza A viruses were prepared in goats (Webster et al., 1974). Post-infection chicken antisera to the isolates from chickens were prepared as described (Palmer et al., 1975). Monoclonal antibodies to the N2 neuraminidase were prepared by the method of Kohler and Milstein (1976) as described by Webster et al., (1982).

RESULTS

Antigenic characterization of Chick/Penn/83 virus

The haemagglutinin (HA) and neuraminidase (NA) of chicken influenza virus isolates were examined serologically to see if antigenic variation had occurred between virus isolated in May 1983 and October 1983 and to examine their relationship to other avian influenza viruses. The chick/-Penn/83 viruses were inhibited to high titres by monospecific antisera to the HA's of A/tern/South Africa/61 and by other antisera to H5 subtypes (table 1). Post-infection chicken antisera showed that the HA of chick/Penn/83 viruses is also related to A/chick/Scotland/59 (H5N2), A/duck/Alberta/57/76 (H5N2) and to A/duck/NY/189/82

(H5N2) but could be distinguished from A/turkey Ontario/-7732/66 (H5N9), A/gull/Md/1756/78 (H5N9) and A/shearwater/-Tryon/624C/75 (H5N3). The HA's of avirulent and virulent chick/Penn/83 viruses were indistinguishable by these polyclonal sera.

TABLE 1   Antigenic Characterization of the Haemagglutinin of Chicken/Pennsylvania/83 Influenza Virus

| Viruses[e] | Haemagglutination inhibition titres with antisera to the following viruses[a] | | | | |
	Dk/Alb/57/75[c]	Tn/SA/61[b]	Sh/Tryon/75[c]	Ty/Ont/66[d]	Ch/Pa/1/83[c]
Dk/Alb/57/76 (H5N2)	320	640	40	160	160
Dk/NY/189/82 (H5N2)	160	320	40	80	80
Tn/SA/61 (H5N3)	160	640	40	40	80
Sh/Tryon/264C/75	160	640	80	160	80
Ty/Ont/7732/66 (H5N9)	<40	320	<40	5120	40
Ch/Scot/59 (H5N1)	640	1280	80	160	320
Ch/Pa/1/83 (H5N2)	160	160	<40	40	640
Ch/Pa/1370/83 (H5N2)	160	320	40	40	640

[a]HI titre is the reciprocal of the highest dilution of antiserum inhibiting 4 haemagglutinating doses of virus
[b]Goat antiserum to isolated H5 HA
[c]Chicken antiserum to intact virus
[d]Rabbit antiserum to intact virus
[e]Viruses inactivated with β-propiolactone

The NA of chick/Penn/83 viruses was inhibited by mono-specific antisera to N2 NA from human isolates in 1957 (table 2). Antisera to the N2 NA of recent human isolates (A/Texas/1/79) did not inhibit the NA activity of chick/Penn/83 viruses. Similarly, the NA from the two chick/Penn/83 viruses were indistinguishable by a panel of monoclonal antibodies to the NA of A/Guiyang/1/57 (H2N2), a 1957 human influenza virus. However, minor antigenic differences could be detected between the chick/Penn/83 viruses and A/Ty/MN/1574/81 (H5N2).

TABLE 2 Characterization of the Neuraminidase on Chicken/
Pennsylvania/83 Influenza Viruses

Neuraminidase inhibition with the following antibodies:

(i) Polyclonal antibodies to:

Viruses	Sing/1/57[a]	Aichi/2/68[b]	Texas/1/79[b]
Guiyang/1/57 (H2N2)	560[c]	230	<50
Texas/1/79 (H3N2)	<50	64	1500
Ty/Mass/3740/65 (H6N2)	1000	<50	<50
Ty/MN/1574/81 (H5N2)	1800	160	<50
Ch(Pa/1/83 (H5N2)	1000	300	<50
Ch/Pa/1370/83 (H5N2)	1000	300	<50

Table 2 cont.

(ii) Monoclonal antibodies to Guiyang/1/57 NA:

	4	11	16	19	31	37	39	40
Guiyang/1/57	8000	2500	5000	5000	2500	600	1000	800
Texas/1/79	-	-	-	-	-	-	-	-
Ty/Mass/3740/65	+[d]	+	+/-	+/-	+	+	+/-	+
Ty/MN/1574/81	+	+/-	-	+	-	+	-	-
Ch/Pa/1/83	+	+	+/-	+/-	+	+	-	+
Ch/Pa/1370/83	+	+	+/-	+/-	+	+	-	+

[a] Goat antiserum to isolated N2 neuraminidase

[b] Rabbit antiserum to intact virus

[c] NI titre = reciprocal of the serum dilution causing 50%
inhibition of virus giving an optical density of 0.50 at
549 nm.

[d]+ = NI titre identical to that obtained with Guiyang/1/57
(H2N2)

+/- = NI titre 4-fold less than that obtained with Guiyang/
1/57 (H2N2)

  - = NI titre at least 10-fold or more less than that
obtained with Guiyang/1/57 (H2N2)

Experimental infection of chickens

Both the early, avirulent chick/Penn/1/83 virus and the
virulent chick/Penn/1370/83 virus infected chickens but the
severity of disease symptoms differed markedly (table 3).
When 10^8 median egg infectious doses (EID_{50}) of the
avirulent viruses were injected intravenously, 75% of
chickens had disease symptoms, there was 38% mortality after
3-5 days and virus could be recovered from all organs of the
dead birds tested, including the brain. All surviving birds
developed high antibody levels. When lower doses (approx.
10^7 EID_{50}) of the avirulent virus were inoculated into the
nasal clefts of chickens, no disease symptoms were detected

(data not presented). However, even lower doses (10^4 EID_{50}) of the virulent virus inoculated into the nasal cleft caused severe symptoms in all chickens, typified by swollen heads, wattles and feet, haemorrhage of the intestinal tract, inability to stand, twisting of the head and 100% mortality within 4-7 days. The birds shed high concentrations of virus in their faeces with up to 10^7 EID_{50}/g being shed from the second day after infection; laying hens continued to produce eggs until the day of death and the last eggs laid by some birds contained high levels of virus in the egg white ($10^{5.6}$ EID_{50}/ml) and yolk ($10^{3.6}$ EID_{50}/ml). Virus transmitted between birds in the same cage and between birds in nearby cages.

TABLE 3   Replication of Chicken/Penn/83 virus in chickens

Virus	Dose (EID_{50})	Route[a]	Virus isolation Tracheal	Rectal	Disease signs	HI antibody
Ch/Pa/1/83	10^8	IV	NA[b]	4/4[c]	3/4 (1 dead)	3/3 (320)[d]
Ch/Pa/1370/ 83	10^4	N	NA	4/4	4/4 (4 dead)	NA

[a]N = nasal, IV = intravenous
[b]NA = not available owing to death of chickens
[c] Number of chickens yielding virus or showing disease symptoms/number exposed. Isolated viruses were identified and shown to be antigenically identical to the inoculated virus.
[d]Figures in parentheses indicate geometric mean titres

These results confirmed that the influenza virus isolated in April 1983 was considerably less virulent for chickens than the virus isolated in October 1983 and that high levels of virus shedding occurred in infected chickens.

Surveillance of man and domestic animals for H5N2 influenza virus

An immediate concern of the influenza task force was whether man was susceptible to the pathogenic chicken virus. Nasal swabs and serum samples were obtained from persons involved with depopulation of chickens and from 110 individuals sampled, two H5N2 isolations were made (table 4). The virus isolations were made from swabs taken immediately after leaving infected chicken houses and virus could not be isolated from the same individuals 12 hours later. Analysis of 109 paired sera showed no antibody rises. These results indicate that man is not susceptible to infection with H5N2 virus but can act as a short term vector.

TABLE 4   Surveillance of man and domestic animals in
          Pennsylvania quarantine zone for H5N2 influenza
          viruses, November 1983-May 1984

Animal Species	Number sampled	Number of influenza virus isolates	Number of H5N2 isolates
Man	110	2	2
Pigs	283	1	1
Ducks	207	0	0
Geese	16	0	0
Peasants	178	0	0
Chuckars	75	1	1
Quail	85	0	0
Turkeys	7	0	0
Peafowl	2	0	0
Total	963	4	4

Many of the infected chicken farms had other domestic animal species. Surveys were carried out to establish whether these species were responsible for H5N2 virus transmission during the outbreak. One H5N2 virus isolate was made from a pig kept in close association with infected chickens (table 4) and another isolation was from a chukar which had apparently escaped depopulation of an infected flock (Nettles et al., 1985). There was also serological evidence of infection in 1.4% of pigs examined (data not presented), which supports the idea that pigs were susceptible to the chicken virus. No influenza viruses were isolated from 346 further domestic gallinaceous birds sampled and from 223 domestic waterfowl sampled although there was serological evidence of infection by viruses containing H5 and N2 surface antigens in 11% of domestic waterfowl (Nettles et al., 1985). This survey suggests that domestic animals did not play a major role in virus transmission during the outbreak.

Surveillance of wild animals for H5N2 virus

There were only 3 influenza virus isolates from 3565 wild animals sampled in Pennsylvania. An H5N1 virus was isolated from a ring-billed gull which had an HA that could be distinguished antigenically from the chicken H5N2 virus. One further H11N1 virus was isolated from a ring-billed gull and an influenza virus, as yet uncharacterized was isolated from a Canada goose. In addition, 18 paramyxoviruses were isolated from avian species during the survey.

TABLE 5 Surveillance of wildlife in Pennsylvania quarantine
zone for H5N2 influenza viruses,
November 1983 - May 1984

Animal Species	Number sampled	Number of Influenza virus isolates	Number of H5N2 isolates
Waterbirds[a]	1275	3[b]	0
Pheasants	84	0	0
Pigeons/doves	480	0	0
Passerines[c]	1426	0	0
Vultures	30	0	0
Rodents[d]	269	0	0
Total	3564	3	0

[a]Comprising ducks, geese, swans and gulls
[b]Two influenza viruses isolated from ring-billed gulls:
 H5N1 and H11N1; one influenza virus from a Canada Goose
 not yet characterized
[c]Comprising crows, starlings, red-wing blackbirds, cowbirds,
 house sparrows, starlings, and other miscellaneous
 passerines
[d]Comprising mice, rats, shrews, muskrats

Although we did not detect H5N2 viruses in wild and domestic pheasants, the National Veterinary Services Laboratory, Ames, Iowa, made a single H5N2 isolation from a hunter-killed ring-necked pheasant (Nettles et al., 1985). It is not known whether the pheasant was wild or was an escaped infected domestic pheasant.

Despite the lack of H5N2 virus isolations from wildlife in Pennsylvania, there was serological evidence that viruses

possessing H5 and N2 surface antigens had been circulating
in 9.6% of the 900 waterbirds sampled. None of the 2,147
non-aquatic birds or rodents tested had detectable
antibodies to H5 or N2 (Nettles et al., 1985).

Although the available evidence suggested that wildlife
were not responsible for H5N2 virus transmission there was
uncertainty about the role of certain animal species in the
outbreak, namely waterfowl, gulls, pheasants and pigs. We
therefore investigated the susceptibility of these species
to experimental infection with virulent H5N2 viruses and
also examined the susceptibility of domestic chickens to
H5N2 viruses circulating in wild ducks and H5N1 virus
circulating in gulls.

Replication of H5N2 viruses in different animal species

Ducks: Experimental infection of ducks with either
avirulent or virulent Chicken/Penn/83 virus demonstrated
biological differences between the chicken viruses and a
typical duck virus. Viruses isolated from wild ducks
normally replicate in cells lining the duck intestine, yet
when inoculated by the tracheal/oral route, the early
chick/Penn/1/83 virus replicated only in the upper
respiratory tract of ducks and the virulent chick/Penn/1370/
83 virus replicated in the intestine of only 1 out of 12
ducks (Table 6). Virus recovered from intestinal replication in ducks was no longer capable of killing chicken
embryos, and it is possible that selection pressures in
ducks had favoured the emergence of an avirulent virus
population. Ducks showing no evidence of virus replication
in trachea or rectum were necropsied, and no virus could be
recovered from faeces, lungs, upper and lower intestine,
bursa, or rectum (data not presented), although there was
serological evidence of infection in all ducks. Neither the
avirulent nor the virulent chick/Penn/83 viruses caused
disease symptoms in ducks. Thus, although ducks were
susceptible to infection with the chicken H5N2 viruses, the
majority of birds failed to shed virus in their faeces.

TABLE 6   Replication of H5N2 viruses in different animal species.

Virus	Dose (EID$_{50}$)	Route[a]	Animal	Virus isolation T/N	R[a]	Disease signs	HI antibody
Ch/Pa/ 1/83	10^4	T/Or	Duck	1/3[b]	0/3	0/3	2/3 (80)
Ch/Pa/ 1370/83	10^8	T/Or	Duck	1/12	1/12	0/12	12/12(905)
Ch/Pa/ 1370/83	10^8	N/Oc	Gull	1/8	0/8	1/8	8/8 (100)
Ch/Pa/ 1370/83	10^7	T/Or	Pheasant	18/18	18/18	7/18	4/4 (905)
Sw/Pa/4 83	10^7	N	Pig	2/2	0/2	2/2[c]	1/2 (80)

a= tracheal, Or = oral, Oc = ocular, N = nasal, R = rectal
b = number yielding virus/number exposed
c = mild coughing that may be unrelated to virus replication

Gulls: since an H5N1 virus was isolated from a ring-billed gull in Pennsylvania during the outbreak the possibility existed that they may also be susceptible to the H5N2 virus.

Ring-billed gulls that had been captured from the wild, were screened for the absence of antibody to H5 influenza haemagglutinin and four days after capture were experimentally infected with the virulent chick/Penn/1370/83 virus by the nasal/ocular route; the same number of gulls were held in quarantine as controls and were not infected. Initially all gulls refused food, and two of eight gulls held in quarantine died with no disease signs. Eight gulls held in containment and infected with the virulent H5N2 virus initially showed no disease signs, and virus was recovered from the trachea of only one of the eight birds (Table 6). One of the infected gulls subsequently died, and virus could be detected in the intestine (10^4 EID_{50}/g), lung, and spleen (10^2 EID_{50}/g). No virus was detected in the brain or other organs. It is not known whether influenza virus infection was responsible for death, for a larger number of uninfected control animals died. Although relatively high concentrations of virus were detected in the intestine, no virus was detected in the faeces. Serological studies showed that all of the surviving gulls produced antibodies to H5N2 virus, indicating that there was limited replication in all of the eight birds inoculated.

Eight seronegative gulls and three chickens placed in cages next to the infected gulls did not become infected and did not seroconvert. Two of the contact gulls died, but there was no evidence of virus infection, and the number of deaths was the same as that in the control group.

These studies demonstrate that although gulls are susceptible to infection with chick/Penn/83 H5N2 influenza virus, only a limited number of birds shed virus and it is not transmissible to either chickens or gulls in adjoining cages.

Pheasants: Eighteen pheasants were experimentally infected with high doses (10^7 EID_{50}) of virulent chick/Penn/-1370/83 virus, and all shed virus in both tracheal and cloacal samples (Table 6). The majority of the pheasants (61%) did not show any signs of disease. The pheasants showing symptoms, became lethargic and dragged their wings but recovered after 2 days. Virus was shed in the faeces ($10^{4.7}$ EID_{50}/g) for up to 15 days after infection. The recovered virus killed chicken embryos within 2 days after inoculation and in this respect was like the virus used to infect the pheasants. All 18 pheasants developed high levels of circulating antibody.

Thus, pheasants were susceptible to infection with the virulent chick/Penn/83 virus and could potentially serve as asymptomatic carriers of virus for long periods.

Pigs: Intranasal inoculation of two young pigs with high concentrations (10^7 EID_{50}) of an H5N2 pig isolate (Swine/Penn/4/83) resulted in virus replication and very mild disease signs. The clinical signs included occasional coughing and splayed back legs, which persisted for 2-3 days. It is not certain whether the mild disease signs were caused by the virus, for no control uninfected pigs were maintained under the same conditions. Virus shedding in nasal secretions (10^3 EID_{50}/ml) persisted for 1-4 days. The infections were not associated with fever, and only one pig developed antibody to the virus. The virus shed in the nasal secretions killed chicken embryos within 3 days of inoculation.

Susceptibility of chickens to H5 viruses circulating in wild birds

The possibility exists that the outbreak of H5N2 virus in chickens in Pennsylvania originated from a virus present in water birds. An H5N2 virus (duck/NY/189/82) isolated from a migratory mallard duck in New York 1 year before the outbreak (Hinshaw et al., 1985) was examined for the ability to infect and cause disease in chickens. After inoculation by the tracheal/oral route, virus could be isolated from the trachea of only one of four birds and was not shed in the faeces of any of the birds (Table 7). The birds showed no disease signs, but they all seroconverted, indicating that limited virus replication had occurred.

Chickens were also inoculated with A/gull/Penn/4175/83 (H5N1), which had been isolated from a ring-billed gull during the Pennsylvania wild life surveillance. This virus gave results similar to those described above for an H5N2 influenza virus from wild ducks: virus replicated in the trachea but not in the cells of the intestinal tract; the chickens showed no disease signs but did seroconvert.

These studies demonstrate that although the H5 viruses isolated from wild ducks and gulls can infect chickens, they

show only limited replication in the upper respiratory tract
and are not shed in the faeces.

TABLE 7 Susceptibility of chickens to H5 viruses from
wild birds

Virus	Dose (EID$_{50}$)	Route[a]	Virus isolation Tracheal	Rectal	Disease signs	HI antibody
Dk/NY/ 189/82 (H5N2)	10^8	T/Or	1/4[b]	0/4	0/4	3/4 (40)
Gull/Pa 4174/83 (H5N1)	10^9	T/Or	2/4	0/4	0/4	3/4 (80)

a = tracheal; Or = oral
b = number of chickens positive/number exposed

DISCUSSION

There is a large influenza virus gene pool maintained
in wild water birds (Hinshaw et al., 1985) and it has been
proposed that these viruses occasionally transmit to
domestic birds and cause outbreaks of disease. There is
evidence for this occurring in domestic turkeys (Halvorson
et al., 1983) and in view of the antigenic similarity
between the chick/Penn/83 virus and H5N2 viruses circulating
in wild ducks in North America over the last 8 years
(Hinshaw et al., 1985) one could speculate that ducks may
have been the original source of the chicken virus.
Wildlife surveillance has failed to demonstrate circulation
of H5N2 virus in wild birds from the quarantine area,
although genetic evidence has confirmed the close
similarities between the chick/Penn/83 virus and viruses

found in wild and domestic birds (Bean et al., 1985).
Furthermore, experimental infections have shown that H5N2
viruses from wild birds can infect chickens although
infections are asymptomatic. It is unlikely that the
chicken H5N2 virus was derived directly from a virulent or
avirulent virus circulating in wild ducks, for both the
early avirulent and later virulent chick/Penn/83 viruses
replicated poorly in ducks, and no virulent virus was shed
in the faeces. This is supported by genetic studies (Bean
et al., 1985) suggesting that the early chick/Penn/83 virus
may have been in the chicken population long enought to
adapt to its new host and change its host specificity.
Alternatively, the original chicken H5N2 virus may be the
result of genetic reassortment between influenza viruses
from wild ducks and gulls and other avian viruses. We
cannot exclude the possibility that the chicken H5N2
influenza virus was derived from another avian species such
as gulls. An H5N1 virus isolated from gulls was able to
infect chickens, although the present studies suggest that
the amount of virus shed in gull faeces was extremely low.

Although we have demonstrated that the avirulent and
virulent chick/Penn/83 viruses are antigenically and geneti-
cally similar (Bean et al., 1985) the HA from the two
viruses can be distinguished by monoclonal antibodies and by
sequence analysis of the HA gene (Kawaoka et al., 1984).
These studies demonstrated that between April and November
1983 there was a change in the gene coding for the HA
affecting a potential glycosylation site which may be
associated with the acquisition of virulence. Another
factor influencing virulence of the H5N2 virus is the
presence of small molecular weight RNA's in the avirulent
virus which may function as defective interfering particles
and modulate the virulence of the early virus (Bean et al.,
1985).

High concentrations of virus were shed in the faeces of
infected chickens which may have provided an excellent
vehicle for virus transmission within and between flocks.

Surveillance of wild life in the quarantine area failed to show evidence of transmission of the H5N2 virus but the present studies have established that ducks, gulls, and pheasants are susceptible to infection with the virulent chick/Penn/1370/83 ihfluenza virus. However, evidence of infection in ducks and gulls was based mainly on serological responses, since virus neither replicated efficiently in the intestine nor was shed in the faeces. Therefore, even if these species were infected in the wild, they were unlikely to have transmitted virus between poultry farms in Pennsylvania. In contrast, pheasants shed virus in faeces for up to 15 days, demonstrating that wild pheasants would be susceptible to the chicken H5N2 influenza virus and could be capable of virus transmission. This possibility is supported by earlier studies by Slemons and Easterday (1972) who reported experimental infection of pheasants with a virulent turkey influenza virus, A/turkey/Ontario/7732/66 (H5N9), and by the isolation of an H5N2 virus from a wild pheasant in Pennsylvania by the National Veterinary Services Laboratory, Ames, Iowa (Nettles et al., 1985). Although the role of pheasants in the introduction or spread of influenza to domestic poultry remains unclear, further surveillance of 84 wild pheasants in the Pennsylvania quarantine area suggests that pheasants were not involved in the Pennsylvania outbreak.

The isolation of an H5N2 virus in a pig exposed to infected poultry in Pennsylvania and the subsequent demonstration of virus replication provides further evidence of transmission of an avian virus to mammals. Avian viruses have been implicated in outbreaks of disease in European pigs (Scholtissek et al., 1983) and in lethal outbreaks of pneumonia in seals off the New England coast (Webster et al., 1981). It is unlikely that pigs transmitted virus during the chick/Penn/83 outbreak, as very few pigs showed evidence of infection despite being in proximity to infected chickens.

These studies have shown that there is a remote chance that wild or domestic animals were involved in virus transmission, but it is more likely that mechanical transmission of virus-laden chicken faeces by humans, flies, or vehicles played a significant part in the transmission of the virus during the outbreak.

The conclusions to be drawn from the Pennsylvania outbreaks may have significant consequences for future, outbreaks of influenza in poultry: 1. As waterbirds continue to harbour an enormous reservoir of influenza viruses, some of which have the potential to cause lethal outbreaks in domestic birds, care should be taken in the housing of domestic birds in order to minimize the chances of contact between wild and domestic birds. 2. Due to the likelihood of mechanical transmission of virus during the outbreak, considerable thought should be given to increased hygiene on poultry farms. 3. There is good evidence that the virulent H5N2 virus emerged from an avirulent virus and consideration should therefore be given to control of both virulent and avirulent influenza outbreaks in poultry. 4. Experimental studies with inactivated H5N2 vaccines (Wood et al., 1985) have provided evidence that vaccination of poultry is effective against lethal chick/Penn/83 virus. Further effort should be directed towards improvement of avian influenza vaccines and consideration given to preparation of vaccine stocks for influenza viruses known to be pathogenic for poultry.

ACKNOWLEDGEMENTS
This work was supported by Cooperative Agreement Number 12-16-93-032 with Emergency Programs, Veterinary Services, Animal and Plant Health Inspection Service, United States Department of Agriculture; The Federal Aid in Wildlife Restoration Act (50 Stat. 917) and Contract Numbers 14-16-0004-83-004 and 14-16-0004-84-005, Fish and Wildlife Service, United States Department of the Interior; grant AI 02649 from the National Institute of Allergy and Infectious Diseases; and by the American Lebanese Syrian Associated Charities. We thank Lisa A. Newberry, Kenneth Cox, Hunter Fleming and Elizabeth Bordwell for excellent technical

assistance. Appreciation is extended to personnel of the
Pennsylvania Game Commission, the Maryland Forest, Park and
Wildlife Service, the Virginia Commission of Game and Inland
Fisheries, the U.S. Fish and Wildlife Service and the
Tennessee Wildlife Resources Agency for their cooperation
and assistance. We are grateful to Dr James Pearson, NVSL,
Ames, for providing virus strains.

REFERENCES

Alexander, D.J. 1982. Avian influenza - recent developments
    Vet. Bull., 52, 341-359.
Bean, W.J., Kawaoka, Y., Wood, J.M., Pearson, J.E. and
    Webster, R.G., 1985. Characterization of virulent and
    avirulent A/chicken/Pennsylvania/83 influenza A viruses:
    potential role of defective interfering RNAs in nature.
    J. Virol., 54, 151-160.
Beaudette, F.R., Hudson, C.B. and Saxe, A.H., 1929. An out-
    break of fowl plaque in New Jersey in 1929. J. Agric.
    Res., 49, 83-92.
Halvorson, D., Karunakaran, D., Senne, D., Kelleher, C.,
    Bailey, C., Abraham, A., Hinshaw, V. and Newman, J.
    1983. Epizootiology of avian influenza-simultaneous
    monitoring of sentinel ducks and turkeys in Minnesota.
    Avian Dis., 27, 77-85.
Hinshaw, V.S., Wood, J.M., Webster, R.G., Deibel, R. and
    Turner, B. (In press). Circulating of influenza viruses
    and para- myxoviruses in waterfowl: comparison of
    different migratory flyways in North America. Bull.
    W.H.O.
Kawaoka, Y., Naeve, C.W. and Webster, R.G., 1984. Is
    virulence of H5N2 influenza viruses in chickens associated
    with loss of carbohydrate from the hemagglutinin.
    Virology, 139, 303-316.
Kohler, G. and Milstein, C., 1976. Derivation of specific
    antibody-producing tissue culture and tumor lines by
    cell fusion. Eur. J. Immunol., 6, 511-519.
Lang, G., Narayan, O., Rouse, B.I., Ferguson, A.E. and
    Connell, M.C., 1968. A new influenza A virus infection
    in turkeys II. A highly pathogenic variant, A/turkey/
    Ontario/7732/66. Canad. Vet. J. 9, 151-160.
Nettles, V.F., Wood, J.M. and Webster, R.G. (In press).
    Wildlife surveillance associated with an outbreak of
    lethal H5N2 avian influenza in domestic poultry. Avian
    Dis.

Palmer, D.F., Coleman, M.T., Dowdle, W.R. and Schild, G.C., 1975. Advanced laboratory techniques for influenza diagnosis. Immunology Series No. 6. U.S. Dept. of Health Education and Welfare.

Scholtissek, C., Burger, H., Bachman, P.A. and Hannoun, C., 1983. Genetic relatedness of hemagglutinins of the HI subtype of influenza A viruses isolated from swine and birds. Virology, 129, 521-523.

Slemons, R.D. and Easterday, B.C., 1972. Host response differences among 5 avian species to an influenza virus - A/Turkey/Ontario/7732/66 (Hav 5 N?). Bull. W.H.O. 47, 521-525.

Webster, R.G., Hinshaw, V.S., Bean, W.J., Van Wyke, K.L., Garaci, J.R. St. Aubin, D.J. and Petursson, G., 1981. Characterization of an influenza A virus from seals. Virology, 113, 712-724.

Webster, R.G., Isachenko, V.A. and Carter, M., 1974. A new avian influenza virus from feral birds in the USSR: recombination in nature? Bull. W.H.O., 51, 324-332.

W.H.O. Report, 1973. Influenza neuraminidase and neuraminidase inhibition procedures. Bull. W.H.O., 48, 199-203.

Wood, J.M., Kawaoka, Y., Newberry, L.A., Bordwell, E. and Webster, R.G. (In press). Standardization of inactivated H5N2 influenza vaccine and efficacy against lethal A/chicken/Pennsylvania/1370/83 infection. Avian Dis.

Wood, J.M., Webster, R.G. and Nettles, V.F., 1985. Host range of A/chicken/Pennsylvania/83 (H5N2) influenza virus. Avian Dis., 29, 198-207.

THE CONTROL AND EPIDEMIOLOGY OF AN INFLUENZA A
OUTBREAK IN IRELAND

T.M. Murphy
Veterinary Research Laboratory
Abbotstown
Castleknock
Dublin 15
Ireland

SUMMARY

An outbreak of avian influenza A/Turkey/Ireland '83 (H5 N8) was contained within a small area and eradicated using the traditional methods of slaughter and burial of infected and in-contact birds. The procedures used in the stamping-out policy are described. Epidemiological surveys failed to identify the initial source of the infection.

INTRODUCTION

Until recently commercial poultry units in Ireland have been free of influenza virus infections. However, in November 1983 an influenza A virus with antigenic determinants H5 N8 and an IVPI 2.83 - 2.85 was isolated from 13 - 18 week old turkeys. Infected birds were depressed, inappetant, diarrhoeic and exhibited nervous signs. Post-mortem examinations revealed an air sacculitis, pericarditis, haemorrhages in the lungs and spleen and duodenitis in the diseased turkeys. Histological studies demonstrated that these birds had a severe encephalitis, with vascular cuffing, neuronal degeneration, foci of gliosis and necrotic changes in the liver, spleen and myocardium. A total of 8000 turkeys on three farms in Co. Monaghan were affected (Table 1). This outbreak of avian influenza represented a serious threat to the poultry industry as the majority of poultry production units are concentrated in the northern counties of Cavan and Monaghan.

TABLE 1   Number of birds and mortalities in depopulated turkey flocks during an influenza A outbreak in Co. Monaghan November/December, 1983.

Holdings	Turkeys		Broilers		Control		
	No. of birds	Deaths	No. of birds	Deaths	Notified	Confirmed	Slaughter
Farm 1	700	400	-	-	21.11.83	28.11.83	-
Farm 11	4700	800	-	-	22.11.83	28.11.83	28.11.83
Farm 111	2600	40	28000	-	30.11.83	2.12.83 (6.12.83)	3.12.83
Farm 1V	120	-	20	-	-	-	28.11.83

Fig. 1 illustrates the epidemic curve. The Central Veterinary Laboratory in Dublin was first alerted to the likelihood of a serious disease in turkeys on 21 November by the local veterinary practitioner. The avian pathologist after inspection of the flocks on Farm I and II advised the veterinary authorities in Dublin and in the local District Veterinary Office (D.V.O., Co. Monaghan) of the possibility of a scheduled (Class A; notifiable disease) poultry disease. A "Disease Outbreak Centre" (DOC) was immediately established in the D.V.O. and Veterinary and Agricultural Officers were deployed in two units, an infected premises unit and a field investigation unit (Fig. 2).

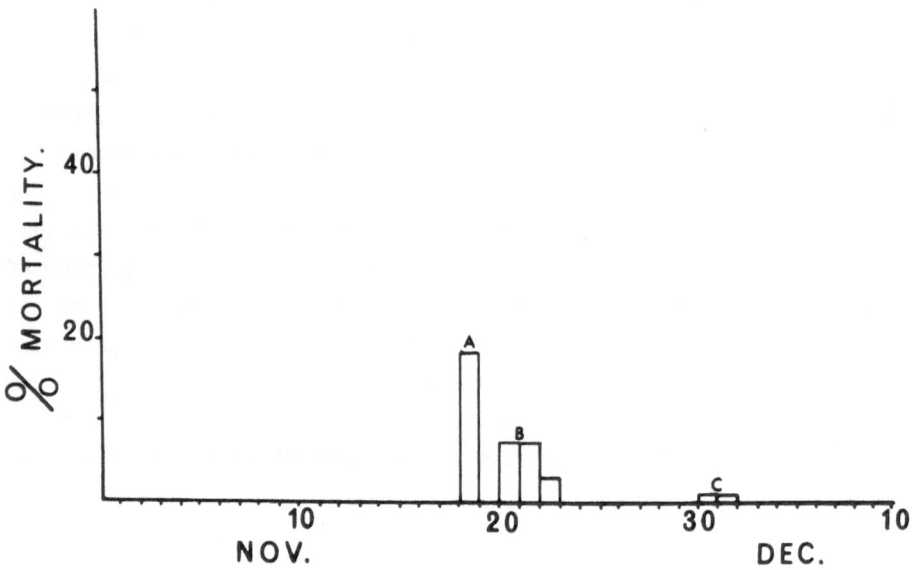

Fig. 1. Epidemic curve of an influenza A/Turkey/Ireland '83 (H5 N8) outbreak in Co. Monaghan Nov./Dec. 1983.
A: Farm 1, B: Farm II, C: Farm III.

```
                    Disease Control Centre
  ┌───────────────────┬───────────────────┬───────────────────┐
  Field               Ante mortem         Infected            Movement
  Investigation       Inspection          Premises            Control
  Unit                Unit                Unit                Co-ordination

  Flock               Onfarm health       Supervision of      Static police
  Visits              investigation       formal restrictions, checks, mobile
  Illness             prior to slaughter  slaughter, carcase  police patrols
  Reports             in meat plant for   and litter disposal,
                      the home market     disinfection
```

Fig. 2.   Deployment of Department of Agriculture officials and police personnel during the influenza A outbreak in Co. Monaghan Nov./Dec. 1983

Movement controls

Following notification that a serious disease outbreak was suspected, formal restrictions were placed on the two turkey farms. All the movement of personnel, live and dead turkeys, poultry feed, litter etc. to and from the farms was prohibited. These restrictions were enforced by the police and Department of Agriculture officials.

A 5km infected zone was established round the infected premises by ministerial order on 29 November. Within this zone all movements of poultry, poultry carcases and hatching eggs were restricted. The holding of poultry sales and hunting of wild fowl was forbidden. These restrictions remained until the end of December. They were imposed by the police who mounted checkpoints at strategic road junctions. The police permitted only those movements authorised by official veterinary personnel attached to the D.O.C. The feed requirements of the non-infected poultry holdings within the "infected zone" were met as required by vehicles operating under official veterinary supervision. The vehicles were subjected to special disinfection procedures.

Slaughter and burial

Slaughter operations on farm II commenced once the presence of avian influenza was confirmed (Table I). The method chosen was manual dislocation of the neck as the houses were old, draughty and in poor condition and unsuitable for the use of gas. Turkeys on farm III were also slaughtered by dislocation of the neck. Chickens in custom built broiler houses on farm III were euthanised with methyl bromide gas at a concentration of $0.45kg/92m^2$.

TABLE 2   Commercial poultry units within the 5km zone of restricted movement.

Production unit	No. of production units	No. of birds	% of bird population in Ireland
Layers	7	39368	1.7
Broilers	13	389300	8.5
Turkeys	24	173650	15.0
Ducks	1	270000	circa 97.0

During the epidemic, serum samples were collected from a representative number of birds in each of the remaining 44 flocks and subjected to the HI test with the specific H5 antigen. All the samples gave a negative response. Poultry flocks in the immediate area outside the 5km zone were also regularly inspected and surveyed for the presence of influenza A virus. A number of flocks were depopulated at this time as the birds were slaughtered for the local Christmas market. These flocks were subjected to a thorough ante-mortem examination on the farm, blood sampling and post-mortem inspection at the point of slaughter.

During the routine epidemiological surveillance operation influenza A virus infection was detected in a large commercial duck unit situated mid-way between farms I and II and within the 5km zone (Table 2). A virus with antigenic determinants H5 N8 was isolated from a large number of 28-34 day old ducks. The majority of birds tested had HI antibodies to the H5 antigen. The IVPI of this duck isolate was similar to the original turkey isolate. This holding was depopulated, carcases, litter and feed etc. was disposed of by burial. The production houses and food stores etc. were cleansed, and disinfected as described for the turkey units. Investigations failed to find any evidence of contact between personnel, vehicles, etc. from the duck farm and the holdings with diseased turkeys.

The carcases, litter (600m^3) and feeding stuffs on all four farms were disposed of by burial. Burial sites were selected on flat ground away from surface water and as close as possible to the poultry houses to avoid disseminating viral material. The prevailing soil type in the area was boulder clay deposited during the ice age. Pits were prepared by heavy plants supplied by the County Council and ranged in size from 240m^3 to 560m^3. All the birds, litter, manure and feeding stuffs were buried at a sufficient depth to ensure 1.2 - 1.5m. covering of soil above them. At least 1.016 tonnes of CaO was placed on the contents of each pit before it was filled in.

Cleansing and disinfection

When a disease outbreak was suspected disinfection commenced on each of the three holdings and continued during the subsequent slaughter and disposal operations. All the areas of the premises including the litter received a preliminary spray with an iodophor disinfectant (Osmodex; Osmonds and Sons Irl. Ltd., dilution 1/80). Once the litter was removed the poultry houses were resprayed with Osmodex using high pressure (675kg/cm^2) washing equipment (Speck-Kolbenpumpen Fabuk, Otto-Speck KG, FGR). The farmyard and other farm buildings were also thoroughly soaked in disinfectant, swept clean and the debris collected and buried.

Surveillance

There were 45 poultry holdings within the 5km restricted movement area (Table 2). These were subjected to daily inspection by a "field investigation unit" (Fig.2). This investigation unit comprised of Veterinary Inspectors and Department of Agriculture poultry personnel not previously exposed to infected birds. Advisory leaflets on disease precautions and clinical signs of illness were distributed to all flock owners within the restricted zone and in the rest of County Monaghan.

The surveillance revealed a suspicious flock (farm III) 1.3km from the original outbreak (Table 1). The turkeys were slaughtered on clinical and histological evidence within 48 hours of notification. Influenza virus was isolated from the tissues of these birds a few days later. Broilers, despite being clinically normal, on the same farm were also slaughtered and destroyed as a precautionary measure. Turkeys on a fourth farm were also slaughtered, as they were considered dangerous contacts, because the flock owner had visited farm II a few days prior to the outbreak.

Epidemiology

The "shoe leather" epidemiological approach of the Veterinary Inspectors in the area failed to pinpoint the original source of the viral infection. Circumstantial evidence suggests that the initial outbreak may have occurred through contact with wild birds. A bird sanctuary is located in the middle of the 5km zone and is inhabited by large numbers of migratory geese and ducks each winter. The breeding ducks on the commercial duck farm were kept on pasture during their rest period between laying seasons. Many of the enclosures were close to a small lake which was populated with wild ducks, gulls, crows and magpies. The turkeys in the three infected holdings were housed in converted farm buildings and no precautions were taken to prevent contact with feral birds. In the case of farm II wild birds on a number of occasions grazed the stubble fields close to the turkey houses. The flock owner of farm I had disposed of the diseased birds by dumping them into a ditch behind the poultry houses. This infected material was a potential source of infection to scavenger birds and the virus may have been disseminated by magpies and starlings. Large numbers of starlings were seen in the turkey houses, feed stores, yard and fields of farm III.

CONCLUSIONS

The influenza outbreak was eradicated fairly quickly by a stamping out policy of slaughter and burial of infected and incontact birds. These measures received commendable support from the flock owners and other sections of the poultry industry. It augurs well for the future that given the co-operation of all sections of the poultry industry any outbreak of a Class A poultry disease can be controlled and eradicated.

ACKNOWLEDGEMENTS

I am indebted to Messrs. J. Moynagh and P. Rogan for assistance with the preparation of this paper.

CURRENT SITUATION OF AVIAN INFLUENZA IN ITALY
AND APPROACHES TO ITS CONTROL

P.N. D'Aprile

Istituto Zooprofilattico Sperimentale delle Venezie
Via G. Orus, 2, 35129 Padova, Italy

ABSTRACT

After a resume of the first cases of avian influenza in Italy, the history of the disease in the last decade is outlined. During this time the predominance for many years of the H6N2 subtype in turkeys was followed by a shift to H9N2 in both chickens and turkeys over the last few years. All isolates proved to be of low pathogenicity and very resistant to pH4. The only report available in the literature about experimental vaccination against Avian Influenza in Italy is summarised and data from experiments still in progress with H6N2 and H9N2 inactivated oil vaccines are presented. The results obtained so far are promising. An indication of the regulatory measures that could be taken for highly pathogenic outbreaks in Italy is described.

INTRODUCTION

Apart from the historical outbreaks of fowl plague from the end of the 18th century to the 1930s, the era of avian influenza began in Italy in 1965 when the late Dr. Rinaldi in collaboration with Dr. Pereira of the WHO Centre in London started a virological survey in Lombardy (North Italy) which led to the isolation of many strains of influenza viruses from chickens, ducks, quails, turkeys and pheasants (Pereira et al., 1967). The majority of these strains were related to the H10N8 subtype, but a few strains belonged to the H6N2 subtype.

In 1967 two strains of H10N8 subtype were also isolated in Veneto (North-eastern Italy) from Japanese quails. The disease was characterized by respiratory symptoms with variable mortalities: up to 75%. Five more strains from quails (H10N8) in Veneto and one from turkeys (unknown subtype) near Naples were isolated from 1969 to 1971 (for references see Petek, 1981).

OUTBREAKS OF THE LAST TEN YEARS

Although the first isolation of influenza virus from turkeys in Veneto was made in 1973, it was not until Dec. 1976 that the disease was observed more frequently in broiler turkeys from the age of 3 months, at first in a narrow area in the province of Verona (Fabris et al., 1977). In the following 3 years the disease spread to most of the province and the bordering provinces, with an increasing number of outbreaks and serologically positive flocks (Franciosi et al., 1981). The outbreaks were observed as a rule in autumn and winter months, but in 1979 the disease was present from January to September. The introduction of stricter hygiene and control measures led to the sudden disappearance of the outbreaks and of serological evidence of infection. The influenza viruses isolated throughout this period were all of the H6N2 subtype.

All turkeys from affected flocks showed sneezing and lacrimation, prostration, anorexia and fever, and sometimes swelling of the infraorbital sinuses with nasal mucous or purulent discharge. The signs lasted about 10 days and mortality varied from 1 to 6%. In animals younger than 3 months the swelling of sinuses reached 40% and mortality reached 20% (Franciosi et al., 1981).

At necropsy, infraorbital sinusitis and seromucous rhinitis were the main findings. Tracheas were congested, sometimes with mucofibrinous plaques. The lungs were often oedematous and sometimes bronchopneumonia was observed. Secondary infections with E. coli and P. multocida were also observed in some outbreaks, and mortality in these cases was greatly increased.

In 1974 the same subtype H6N2 was isolated in Lombardy from turkeys. In the same region, during a survey on migratory birds a H10N8 strain was isolated from a swallow in 1977, although all isolation attempts from other birds were negative. In 1979 an H6N2 strain was isolated in Emilia region from guinea fowls.

In 1980 influenza outbreaks were sporadic. An isolation of H6N6 subtype was made from turkeys in the province of Verona where H6N2 subtype was previously prevalent. One more outbreak in turkeys led to the isolation of an H5N2 subtype in the province of Bergamo (Lombardy), and the same subtype was isolated from hens with a drop in egg production in the same province. The H10N8 subtype, prevalent from 1965, was again isolated from quails in 1980 (Petek, 1981).

No isolations were made in 1981 and no serological evidence of infection was found in a survey on 200 turkey flocks. In 1982 a single strain of H6N2 subtype was isolated in the province of Verona. In the same year an H7N2 subtype was isolated in the province of Ferrara (Emilia) from turkey hens with a drop in egg production (Cirelli, 1984).

In 1983 the disease spread to the whole Veneto Region, mostly in turkeys from 20 to 60 days old with an acute respiratory syndrome and sometimes with diarrhoea. Infraorbital sinusitis, seromucous rhinitis and tracheitis were the common findings at necropsy with no other character- istic lesions. The symptoms lasted about 10 days and the mortality was about 2%. In cases with secondary bacterial infections, mortality reached 10-15%, especially in younger birds (Cirelli, 1984). Five strains from these outbreaks were of H9N2 subtype and one of H6N1.

In 1984 two H6 and one H9 isolations were made (the neuraminidase has not yet been typed), all in the province of Verona from outbreaks in turkeys from 10 to 16 weeks old, with the symptoms described above. One isolation of H9 subtype was made in the same province from 40 day old chickens which showed prostration, cyanotic comb and wattles and ataxia. A common finding in all outbreaks was enteritis with a greenish colour of the intestinal contents. So far in 1985 two isolations have been made, both from chickens in the province of Verona. The symptoms were as before, and in one outbreak (in the same farm of the outbreak observed in 1984) a drop in egg production from 70 to 20% was observed. In both cases the haemagglutinin was H9.

The intravenous pathogenicity indices of 9 strains of H6N2 and one strain of H6N1 virus isolated from 1973 to 1983 were always very low, never exceeding 0.21 (Table 1). For one strain H6N2 the intranasal in-contact pathogenicity test was performed in two weeks old turkeys, and the indices were 0.7 for infected birds and 0.5 for in-contact birds (Table 1) (Franciosi et al., 1981). None of these strains produced plaques in chick- en embryo fibroblasts in the absence of trypsin.

TABLE 1   Pathogenicity Indices

	IVPI in 6 weeks old chickens	
turkey/Italy/1973-79	6 strains H6N2	0.00*
turkey/Italy/78	H6N2	0.15*
turkey/Italy/82	2 strains H6N2	0.00
turkey/Italy/83	H6N1	0.21
	INCPI in 2 weeks old turkeys	
turkey/Italy/76	H6N2	IN 0.7*
		C 0.5*

* data from Franciosi et al. (1981).

Most of the isolates were tested for their resistance to pH 4.
(Table 2). Of 14 H6N2 strains, 11 lost less than 1 log infectivity and
only one reached a loss of 2.8 log. The two H6N1 and H6N6 strains both
lost 1 log infectivity and the two H5N2 strains lost less than 1 log,
whereas the H7N2 strain lost 3.6 log. Strains of the H10N8 subtype from
ducks and quails lost from 2.5 to 4.8 log, the H9 strains from turkeys and
chickens tested to date lost from 1.0 to 2.2 log, and the two new H6

TABLE 2   Sensitivity to pH 4 (10 minutes at 4°C)*

Avian strains isolated in Italy (1965-83)		
turkey/Italy/1976-82	11 strains H6N2	0.0-0.8
chicken/Italy/80	H5N2	0.6
turkey/Italy/80	H5N2	0.8
turkey/Italy/80	H6N6	1.0
turkey/Italy/83	H6N1	1.0
guinea fowl/Italy/79	H6N2	1.4
turkey/Italy/76	H6N2	1.8
quail/Italy/67	H10N8	2.4
turkey/Italy/80	H6N2	2.8
turkey/Italy/77	H10N2	3.4
turkey/Italy/82	H7N2	3.6
duck/Italy/65	2 strains H10N8	3.4-4.4
quail/Italy/70	H10N8	3.8
quail/Italy/79	H10N8	4.8
More recent isolates		
turkey/Italy/83	H9N?	2.2
turkey/Italy/84	2 strains H6N?	0.0-0.6
turkey/Italy/84	H9N?	1.0
chicken/Italy/84	H9N?	1.6
Other strains for comparison		
parrot/Ulster/73	H7N1	2.8
Singapore/57	H2N2	3.2
horse/Italy/81	H3N8	3.4
duck/England/56	H11N6	4.6
Victoria/75	H3N2	5.6
WSN/33	H1N1	6.4

* expressed as log EID_{50} (pH 7.0)- log EID_{50} (pH 4.0).
  Data partly taken from Petek and D'Aprile (1980).

isolates not yet completely typed lost less than 1 log infectivity (Petek
and D'Aprile, 1980). These findings suggest that these low virulent H6
and H9 strains could be at a selective advantage by their resistance in the
environment. It is also noteworthy that the H6N2 subtype could be isolated
from the faeces 60 days after the beginning of the symptoms. This obviously does not rule out the possibility that the subtype could be carried

yearly in the area by water-fowl, but direct evidence for this is lacking since no virological survey on water-fowl has recently been undertaken.

APPROACHES TO THE CONTROL OF INFLUENZA

Until now there is only one report, by Dr. Zanella at the Symposium on Avian Influenza held in Beltsville, Maryland in 1981, dealing with experimental vaccination of turkeys and chickens in Italy. This author vaccinated groups of 3 week old SPF chickens and commercial turkeys with an avian influenza and Newcastle disease combined vaccine, both viruses inactivated with Betapropiolactone and emulsified with 70% mineral oil. The subtypes of influenza virus used were H6N2, H5N2, and H10N2. The HI response was quite low, particularly in turkeys after a single dose of vaccine, whereas the second vaccination after 3-4 weeks raised the HI titres to good levels. A good protection was achieved against the homologous serotype after challenge, but very low or no cross-protection was induced (in terms of reisolation of the virus after challenge) by the other viruses with different H antigens but all containing the same N2 antigen. The author emphasised the importance of the availability of polyvalent vaccines, of the determination of the subtypes involved at times, and the monitoring of the antibody spectrum in big integrated farms and in areas with a high concentration of birds (Zanella et al., 1981).

Another series of experiments is now being performed by our group. Groups of 20 two week old chickens were vaccinated with inactivated vaccine (Betapropiolactone 0.1% for two hours at 37°C) emulsified with 75% mineral oil. The birds received 160 HAU each in 0.5 ml vaccine by the subcutaneous route. One group was vaccinated with H6N2 subtype, another group with H9 N2 and a third group with both (160 + 160 HAU); half of each group was revaccinated 3 weeks after the first vaccination with the same amount of viruses.

Hemagglutination inhibition tests were performed at weekly intervals, and the results obtained to date, expressed as geometric mean titres, are shown in Table 3.

From the data it is apparent that quite a good booster effect is obtained in revaccinated groups, although in non-revaccinated groups increasing levels of HI antibodies are also observed until the 6th week post vaccination, in accordance with the theory that second vaccination would not be required when a good vaccine is used. Also interesting is the fact

TABLE 3 Geometrical mean titres of HI in groups of 10 vaccinated chickens.

Vaccines	HI with H6N2 virus at weekly intervals					
	1	2	3	4	5	6
H6N2	1	26.36	85.74	85.74	171.48	226.25
H6N2 ✳	0	18.24	59.29	105.56	183.79	367.28
H6N2+H9N2	0	12.61	40.00	40.00	103.75	207.49
H6N2+H9N2✳	0	18.24	42.87	64.98	160.00	342.77
	HI with H9N2 virus at weekly intervals					
H9N2	0	8.18	18.06	23.33	54.43	58.79
H9N2✳	0	11.23	34.82	34.82	52.78	138.28
H6N2+H9N2	0	17.14	24.38	14.99	32.71	123.31
H6N2+H9N2 ✳	0	13.18	28.28	22.97	80.00	211.10

✳ Revaccinated 3 weeks after the 1st vaccination.

that the response of H9N2 virus, not very immunogenic in itself, is enhanced in the group treated with the combined vaccines, even with a single vaccination (as judged from the results at 6 weeks post inoculation). The practical impact of these results would be obviously better evaluated after challenge experiments have been carried out.

As to regulatory measures for outbreaks of avian influenza caused by highly pathogenic strains, the Italian Health Ministry would be oriented towards a slaughter policy combined with ring vaccination. Indeed, a meeting was held in Rome in which some isolates were chosen with H5 and H7 haemagglutinins for the production of an inactivated emulsified polyvalent vaccine, but as yet the production has not started although the growth characteristics of strains involved have already been studied.

At a recent meeting of the Italian Society of Avian Pathology, Dr. Barret Cowen of the Pennsylvania State University stressed the suitability of vaccination against both low and high pathogenic influenza viruses with inactivated vaccines, on the basis of the experience of 6 years of vaccination in turkeys in the USA. In particular he pointed out the lack of evidence for an increased probability of drifting of avirulent viruses to a highly virulent form in presence of vaccination, and stressed the fact that a slaughter policy is too costly even for countries like the United States (Cowen et al., 1985).

This theory is likely to be the subject of much discussion in the future among avian pathologists and representatives of the Ministry of Health.

REFERENCES

Cirelli, L. 1984. Andamento dell'influenza aviaria negli allevamenti di tacchini del Veneto. Riv. Avicol., 53, 5, 33-35.
Cowen, B.S., Wilson, R.A. and Braune, M.O. 1985. Simposio della Soc. It. di Patol. Aviare sull'Influenza aviare, Milano, Italia, 6/6/1985.
Fabris, G., Cabasso, E. and Allodi, C. 1977. Alcuni aspetti e problemi legati alla presenza di E. coli in sindromi respiratorie dei tacchini. La Clinica Vet. 100, 448-459.
Franciosi, C, D'Aprile, P.N., Alexander, D.J. and Petek, M. 1981 Influenza A virus infections in commercial turkeys in North East Italy. Avian Pathol., 10, 303-311.
Pereira, H.G., Rinaldi, A. and Nardelli, L. 1967. Antigenic variation among avian influenza A viruses. Bull. WHO, 37, 553-567.
Petek, M. 1981. Current situation in Italy. Proc. 1st Symp. on Avian Influenza, Beltsville, Maryland, 31-34.
Petek, M. and D'Aprile, P.N. 1980. Sensitivity to pH4 of different strains of Influenza A. Microbiologica, 3, 471-474.
Zanella, A., Poli, G. and Bignami, M. 1981. Avian Influenza: approaches to the control of disease with inactivated vaccines in oil emulsion. Proc. 1st Symp. on Avian Influenza, Beltsville, Maryland, 180-183.

AVIAN INFLUENZA: DIAGNOSIS AND VACCINATION

M.S. McNulty, J.B. McFerran

Veterinary Research Laboratories, Stormont, Belfast BT4 3SD,
Northern Ireland

ABSTRACT

Direct immunofluorescent staining of tissue impression smears is a rapid, specific diagnostic test for avian influenza, which is as sensitive as virus isolation in chick embryos. A FITC-conjugated antiserum prepared against one subtype of influenza virus stains antigenically unrelated subtypes. Diagnosis by inoculation of chick cell cultures is insensitive compared with immunofluorescence or embryo inoculation.

The protection induced in chickens by live neuraminidase (N)-specific vaccines against challenge with highly pathogenic avian influenza viruses was investigated. Vaccination with viruses belonging to N1 and N8 subtypes conferred protection against challenge with viruses of the same N subtype and irrelevant haemagglutinin (H) subtypes. A particular advantage of N-specific vaccines is that they do not interfere with serological diagnosis by haemagglutination inhibition tests. The anomalous cross-protection between viruses of H1 and H5 subtypes could be exploited to control outbreaks of disease caused by highly pathogenic H5 viruses by using vaccines based on H1 and the appropriate N antigen.

INTRODUCTION

A devastating outbreak of avian influenza (AI), involving over 17 million birds, occurred in 1983/4 in the USA, principally in Pennsylvania and Virginia. This outbreak was unusual in several respects. Firstly, the disease occurred predominantly in chickens, whereas most previous outbreaks have been in turkeys. Secondly, having initially caused a relatively mild disease in layer and broiler flocks over a period of about 6 months, the virus appeared to show a sudden increase in pathogenicity. Thirdly, the disease spread rapidly over a wide area. In most previously described outbreaks of highly pathogenic avian influenza (HPAI), there was very little spread and the outbreaks tended to be self-limiting.

An outbreak of HPAI occurred in turkeys in the Republic of Ireland in 1983 (Anon, 1984; McNulty et al., 1985a). This was successfully and quickly eradicated by slaughter by the veterinary authorities in the Republic. However, in view of the American experience and the highly unpredictable occurrence of outbreaks in domestic poultry, we initiated work to ensure that we would be able to deal effectively with future outbreaks of AI, whether rapidly spreading or not. Results of current studies on two key areas, namely diagnosis and vaccination, are summarised in this paper.

DIAGNOSIS

Laboratory diagnosis of AI is based on (a) isolation, antigenic sub-typing and pathotyping of the virus and/or (b) detection of antibodies to the virus. The standard method for virus isolation is to inoculate each clinical specimen into five or six 9-11 day old chicken embryos via the allantoic route. Normally a minimum incubation period of 2 days is requir-ed before death of embryos is observed. However if no haemagglutinin is produced during the first passage in chick embryos, or if haemagglutination titres are insufficient to allow identification of the virus, a second passage in embryos is required (Beard, 1975). This procedure is time-consuming, laborious and costly, and imposes considerable strain on lab-oratory resources when required to deal with the influx of specimens which occurs during a large outbreak.

We have investigated the use of direct immunofluorescence as a screen-ing test for detecting AI virus in tissue specimens. The main findings, which have been published in detail elsewhere (Allan and McNulty, 1985), are described below.

Impression smears of organs and tissues were made on degreased glass microscope slides, air-dried, fixed in acetone for 10 minutes at room temperature and stained for 1 hour at 37°C with FITC-conjugated antisera to AI virus, which had been prepared in chickens or ducks.

It was found that antisera prepared by immunizing birds with a par-ticular subtype of AI virus were capable of detecting antigens of AI virus-es belonging to the same and different subtypes. However, generally speak-ing, brighter staining was obtained with homologous antisera. This was reflected in the titres of the conjugated antisera determined using dif-ferent antigens eg the titres of a conjugated antiserum to A/duck/England/ 56 (H11 N6) virus using material infected with the homologous virus and with A/chicken/Scotland/59 (H5 N1) virus were 1:320 and 1:40 respectively. However, highest titres were obtained with a conjugated polyvalent anti-serum prepared by immunizing chickens with three different subtypes of AI virus.

Using material from chickens experimentally infected with avirulent and highly pathogenic AI viruses, results of diagnosis by direct immuno-fluorescence were compared with those obtained by virus isolation in chicken embryos and chick cell cultures.

Using fresh material there was a good correlation between the results obtained by direct immunofluorescence and virus isolation in chick embryos. Of 89 specimens examined, 41 were positive by both tests, 44 were negative by both tests, 2 were positive by immunofluorescence and negative by virus isolation and 2 were positive by virus isolation and negative by immuno-fluorescence. However, virus isolation was unsuccessful in the case of a bird that had been left for 4 days at room temperature before necropsy, although positive immunofluorescence was detected in brain, conjunctival and kidney smears. In most positive tissue impression smears, large numbers of fluorescing cells were present. Most showed diffuse cyto-plasmic staining with small inclusions (Fig. 1), occasional cells also had nuclear fluorescence.

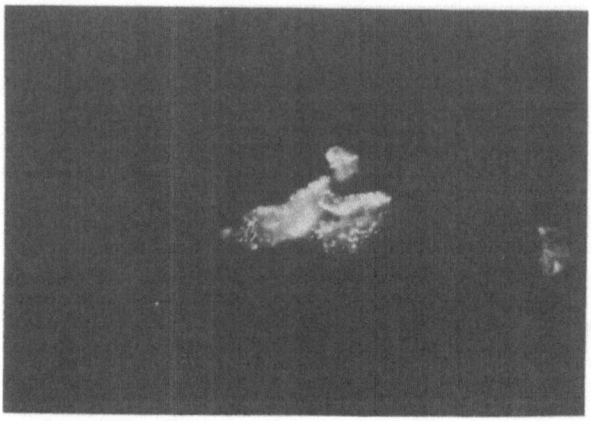

Fig. 1   Immunofluorescent staining of influenza virus antigens in tracheal impression smear.

The choice of specimens to be examined by immunofluorescence is largely dictated by the presenting clinical signs and gross pathological findings. If birds are showing respiratory signs, conjunctiva, trachea and lung should obviously be examined. Any visceral organs showing gross changes should also be examined.

Chick cell cultures have obvious attractions in terms of more econ-omical use of eggs than embryo inoculation. However, virus isolation in cell cultures was less successful than isolation in chick embryos. Only 4 isolates were made in chick embryo fibroblasts from 52 specimens from which virus was isolated using chick embryos. Using chick embryo liver cells 23 isolates were made from the same specimens. In addition to poor sensitivity, other problems are encountered with isolation in cell cultures. In general, about 5 days incubation in cell cultures are required before growth of the virus can be detected by either c.p.e. or haemagglutination. Furthermore, reoviruses and adenoviruses grow well in chick embryo liver cell cultures. This can be troublesome, particularly with specimens from broilers, which have a high prevalence of infections with these viruses, as growth of reovirus and adenovirus may mask the growth of influenza virus.

The following conclusions and comments can be made from this work.

1. Direct immunofluorescent staining of tissue impression smears is as sensitive as chick embryo inoculation for detecting AI virus. Immuno- fluorescence has some advantages over embryo inoculation. It is quicker, results can be available within 2 hours. It is specific, whereas a number of different viruses can kill embryos and haemagglut- inate.

2. Direct immunofluorescence is particularly useful as a rapid screening test. This has obvious applications in an outbreak situation ie to identify infected flocks or to quickly eliminate influenza as the cause of any unexplained increase in mortality.

3. A disadvantage is that one has still to isolate the virus from material showing positive immunofluorescence. However immunofluorescence will identify those organs which contain the greatest amounts of antigen, thereby decreasing the number of specimens which need to be inoculated into chick embryos. Immunofluorescence results may be a guide to the pathogenicity of an influenza virus. HPAI viruses tend to invade most of the body systems, while low pathogenic strains tend to be more localized.

4. A conjugated antiserum prepared against one subtype of influenza virus stains other antigenically unrelated subtypes.

5. The use of chick cell cultures cannot be recommended as a sensitive system for primary isolation of AI viruses.

VACCINATION

In spite of the economic significance of AI, comparatively little work has been done on vaccination against the disease. Of the two surface antigens of the virus, the haemagglutinin (H) is generally believed to be more important than the neuraminidase (N) in terms of conferring immunity (Alexander, 1982; Brugh et al., 1979). Thus inactivated vaccines have generally incorporated either the currently prevalent strains or H subtypes (Eskelund, 1984). However this interferes with serological diagnosis by HI tests, in that it is impossible to distinguish vaccinal antibody from antibody arising from a field challenge. Rott et al. (1974) demonstrated that antibody to the N antigen plays a significant role in the development of immunity to AI. We have examined the possibility of protecting chickens against challenge with HPAI viruses by using model, live N-specific vaccines ie vaccines incorporating viruses of the same N subtype but different H antigens from the challenge virus. The results of this work (McNulty et al., 1985b) are summarized below.

Two non-pathogenic AI viruses, A/parrot/Ulster/73 (H7 N1) and A/duck/Alberta/35/76 (H1 N1) and an equine influenza virus A/equine/Miami/1/63 (H3 N8) were used as vaccines. These were administered by intranasal and intraconjunctival installation, intramuscular inoculation or via the drinking water (Table 2). Commercial broilers or SPF White Leghorn chickens between 1 and 7 weeks of age were vaccinated twice, at an interval of 2-3 weeks and challenged about 2 weeks after the second vaccination. The following HPAI viruses were used as challenge strains: A/chicken/Scotland/59 (H5 N1), A/turkey/England/63 (H7 N3) and A/turkey/Ireland/83 (H5 N8). All viruses were grown in chick embryos and undiluted infected allantoic fluid was used to vaccinate and challenge the birds. Challenge virus was inoculated directly onto the nasal passages and conjunctival sac of each bird (direct challenge) or directly challenged unvaccinated controls were placed in contact with vaccinated birds (indirect challenge). In each experiment unvaccinated controls and vaccinates were housed together in the same air and floor space.

A cross-protection experiment designed to confirm the protective capacity of antibody to the 2 surface antigens of the virus (Allan et al., 1971; Rott et al., 1974) was carried out (Table 1). Chickens were vaccinated by intranasal, intraconjunctival and oral administration of parrot/Ulster (H7 N1) virus and challenged directly with chick/Scotland/ (H5 N1) or turkey/England (H7 N3) viruses. Vaccinates remained healthy, while 75-100% of unvaccinated controls died. Vaccinates were given a second challenge, this time with turkey/Ireland (H5 N8) virus. Vaccinates previously challenged with chick/Scotland (H5 N1) virus had developed antibody to H5 and remained healthy. However vaccinates previously challenged with turkey/England (H7 N3) virus were not protected against the second challenge.

TABLE 1   Cross-protection experiment.

Vaccine	1st Challenge	2nd Challenge
	turkey/England (H7 N3)	turkey/Ireland (H5 N8)
	0/11 vaccinates died 3/4 controls died	9/11 vaccinates died 3/4 controls died
parrot/Ulster (H7 N1)		
	chick/Scotland (H5 N1)	turkey/Ireland (H5 N8)
	0/10 vaccinates died 4/4 controls died	0/10 vaccinates died 4/4 controls died

This experiment showed that prior exposure to viruses possessing either the same H or N antigens as the challenge virus conferred protection against challenge, confirming the findings of Allan et al. (1971) and Rott et al. (1974). The non-protective nature of antibody to the internal antigens of the virus (Allan et al., 1971) was also demonstrated.

Experiments investigating the ability of chickens vaccinated in different ways with N-specific vaccines to withstand direct or indirect challenge with HPAI viruses were also performed (Table 2). These showed that protection could be induced by vaccination with viruses possessing the same N subtype and different H subtype from the challenge virus. Thus vaccination with H7 N1 or H1 N1 protected against challenge with H5 N1 and vaccination with H3 N8 conferred protection against H5 N8.

The protection in Experiment 4 can be partially attributed to antibody to H1. Alexander and Parsons (1980) have demonstrated an anomalous relationship between H1 and H5. Although H1 and H5 appear to be antigenically distinct, chickens previously exposed to viruses of H1 subtype were partially protected against challenge with H5 HPAI viruses. The existence of a similar anomalous relationship between H7 and H5 appears to be ruled out by failure of vaccination with H7 N1 to protect against challenge with H5 N8 (Experiment 5). Similarly the failure of H3 N8 to protect against challenge with H5 N1 (Experiment 6) shows that the protection afforded against H5 N8 by vaccination with H3 N8 (Experiment 5) is not mediated through an anomalous relationship between H3 and H5.

The following conclusions and comments can be made from these experiments.

1. N-specific vaccines are efficacious in protecting chickens against

TABLE 2. Summary of Vaccination Experiments

Experiment No.	Vaccine Virus	Route of Administration	Challenge Virus	Type of challenge	Survival of Vaccinates	Controls
2	parrot/Ulster (H7N1)	Drinking water x 2	chick/Scotland (H5N1)	Direct	39/54 (72%)	1/20 (5%)
3	parrot/Ulster (H7N1)	i/nasal, i/conj x 2	chick/Scotland (H5N1)	Indirect	21/21 (100%)	3/10 (30%)
4	duck/Alberta (H1N1)	i/nasal, i/conj x 1; i/musc x 1	chick/Scotland (H5N1)	Direct	23/23 (100%)	0/10 (0%)
5	equine/Miami (H3N8)	i/musc x 2	turkey/Ireland (H5N8)	Direct	20/25 (80%)	0/10 (0%)
	or parrot/Ulster (H7N1)	i/nasal, i/conj x 1; i/musc x 1			1/20 (5%)	
6	equine/Miami (H3N8)	as expt 5	chick/Scotland (H5N1)	Direct	8/24 (33%)	2/10 (20%)
	or parrot/Ulster (H7N1)	as expt 5			9/9 (100%)	

challenge with HPAI viruses.

2. We used live virus vaccines as a convenient model system. It seems unlikely that the use of live influenza vaccines would be permitted in poultry (Alexander, 1982). Therefore this work needs to be repeated with inactivated vaccines. However, as two of the viruses used as vaccines, duck/Alberta (H1 N1) and equine/Miami (H3 N8) did not appear to grow in chickens and had to be given parenterally to stimulate a significant immune response, there is no reason to believe that in-activated vaccines should not also be efficacious.

3. The main advantage of N-specific vaccines is that they do not inter-fere with serological diagnosis by HI tests. It is possible by HI testing to distinguish between vaccinated flocks which have received a field challenge and those which have not. This counters one of the main arguments against vaccination.

4. While eradication by slaughter will remain the measure of choice to deal with outbreaks of AI, N-specific vaccines could be used to ring vaccinate around an eradication area. A policy of slaughter and ring vaccination was successfully used in 1973 in Northern Ireland to control airborne velogenic Newcastle disease.

5. The anomalous relationship between H1 and H5 subtypes could be ex-ploited to control outbreaks caused by H5 subtype viruses, by using vaccines based on H1 and the appropriate neuraminidase. This re-lationship is particularly fortuitous because all outbreaks of HPAI described to date have been caused by either H5 or H7 subtypes.

REFERENCES

Alexander, D.J. 1982. Avian influenza - recent developments. Vet. Bull., 52, 341-359.

Alexander, D.J. and Parsons, G. 1980. Protection of chickens against challenge with virulent influenza A viruses of Hav 5 subtype con-ferred by prior infection with influenza A viruses of Hsw 1 subtype. Arch. Virol., 66, 265-269.

Allan, G.M. and McNulty, M.S. 1985. A direct immunofluorescence test for the rapid detection of avian influenza virus antigen in tissue im-pression smears. Avian Path., in Press.

Allan, W.H., Madeley, C.R. and Kendal, A.P. 1971. Studies with avian in-fluenza A viruses: Cross protection in chickens. J. gen. Virol., 12, 79-84.

Anonymous. 1984. Bull, Int. Off. Epizootics, 96, 22.

Beard, C.W. 1975. Avian influenza. In "Isolation and Identification of avian Pathogens" (Ed. S.B. Hitchner, C.H. Domermuth, H.G. Purchase and J.E. Williams). (American Association of Avian Pathologists, New York).

Brugh, M., Beard, C.W. and Stone, H.D. 1979. Immunization of chickens and turkeys against avian influenza with monovalent and polyvalent oil emulsion vaccines. Am. J. Vet. Res., 40, 165-169.

Eskelund, K.E. 1984. Use of inactivated vaccine to control avian influenza outbreaks. Proc. 33rd West. Poult. Dis. Conf., 8-10.

McNulty, M.S., Allan, G.M., McCracken, R.M. and McParland, P.J. 1985a. Isolation of a highly pathogenic influenza virus from turkeys. Avian Path., 14, 173-176.

McNulty, M.S., Allan, G.M. and Adair, B.M. 1985b. Efficacy of avian influenza neuraminidase - specific vaccines in chickens. Avian Path., in Press.

Rott, R., Becht, H. and Orlich, M. 1974. The significance of influenza virus neuraminidase in immunity. J. gen. Virol., 22, 35-41.

EXPERIMENTAL VACCINATION OF CHICKENS AGAINST
AVIAN INFLUENZA SUBTYPE H5 WITH AN
INACTIVATED OIL EMULSION VACCINE

B. Kouwenhoven and A.G. Burger

Poultry Health Institute
P.O. Box 43, 3940 AA DOORN
The Netherlands

ABSTRACT

Doses of 500, 125 or 62.5 μl of two inactivated influenza vaccines prepared using the virulent A/tern/S. Africa/61 (H5N2) strain were injected subcutaneously into five week old SPF chicks.

HI antibody appeared faster but also waned faster after vaccination with vaccine A, in aqueous solution, than with the oil emulsion based vaccine B. This was associated with a slightly better protection against challenge with the virulent live virus by vaccine A 3 weeks after vaccination. Challenge was not followed by a significant increase of HI titres or appearance of precipitating antibody. Virus titres were approximately the same in faecal samples from all vaccinated groups and from a non-vaccinated control group at the third day after challenge.

Birds had higher mean HI titres 11 weeks after vaccination with vaccine B than with vaccine A, and were better protected against challenge. An increase in HI titres and the appearance of precipitating antibody was observed after challenge of the less well protected groups vaccinated with 500 or 125 μl of vaccine A.

While most birds that died or became sick had no circulating antibody at the time of challenge, some had titres of 3, 4 or 5. However, many vaccinated birds without circulating antibody overcame challenge without developing symptoms.

INTRODUCTION

Although in case of an influenza outbreak an eradication policy would be followed to control the disease in The Netherlands, it was necessary to know to what extent vaccination with an inactivated vaccine against influenza serotype H5 would result in protection.

We were interested in the potency of such a vaccine with respect to production of circulating antibody, protection against mortality and morbidity and to virus recovery after challenge with a virulent virus. The strain A/tern/S. Africa/61 (H5N2) was chosen as a challenge virus since it causes a high morbidity and mortality. The disadvantage of this strain is that while it grows to high titres, it produces only low titres of haemagglutinin (HA). Two vaccine formulations (A and B) were tested. B was known to stimulate high haemagglutination inhibition (HI) titres in turkeys with another subtype of influenza virus. Vaccine A, an aqueous solution, was expected to stimulate an earlier but not a higher antibody response than vaccine B.

MATERIALS AND METHODS

Vaccine preparation

The A/tern/S. Africa/61 influenza virus was propagated in SPF chicken eggs. Eggs were inoculated in the allantoic cavity at day 9 or 10 of incubation; all embryos had died within 24 h. The allantoic fluids of the individual eggs were pooled, clarified by centrifugation at 3000 g for 10 minutes and tested for bacteriological sterility.

The HA titre of the pool was 1:64 and the virus titre measured by titration in hatching eggs was $10^{8.5}$ ELD_{50} per 0.2 ml.

The virus in one litre of this suspension was inactivated at room temperature by adding (dropwise during 15 minutes) diluted reagent grade formalin to 0.445% final concentration. The suspension was stirred in a sterile Erlenmeyer flask during the addition of formalin. Stirring was continued for a further 5 minutes after the last formalin had been added. Thereafter the suspension was transferred to another sterile Erylenmeyer flask and left for 24 h at room temperature whereupon it was kept at + 4°C.

Inactivation was controlled by inoculation of 0.2 ml of the suspension into the allantoic cavity of each of 30 ten days incubated SPF eggs. Although embryos dying within 24 h were regarded as non-specific, their allantoic fluids were tested for absence of HA activity. The allantoic fluids from embryos that had eventually died up to 96 h p.i. and those from the surviving embryos were harvested separately and inoculated into another series of 10 days incubated eggs. The allantoic fluids from the latter were tested for absence of HA activity 96 h later. The influenza virus appeared to be inactivated.

Vaccines A and B were made from the inactivated suspension by incorporation into the appropriate adjuvants and emulsion. The antigen concentration in the finished products was 10 per cent by volume.

Experimental design

Three groups of 30 five week old SPF chicks were injected individually in the neck with 500, 125, 62.5 µl of vaccine A. Three other groups of 30 birds were injected similarly with vaccine B. Birds were housed in an isolated pen together with 30 non-vaccinated birds.

Blood was collected from 15 individual birds for determination of HI antibodies 1, 2, 3, 5, 7 and 9 weeks after vaccination. HI titrations were performed essentially as described for Newcastle disease virus by De Jong (1978) using 8 HA units of antigen.

Three weeks after vaccination 15 birds from each vaccinated group and 15 control birds were placed in each of 7 isolators and challenged by ocular instillation of $10^{5.3}$ ELD_{50} virus per bird. Birds were observed daily for clinical symptoms and mortality during 2 weeks. Three days after this challenge, fresh faeces was collected for virus isolation from all individual birds in isolator 7 (not vaccinated but challenged birds) that had survived up to that time as well as from an equal number in the other groups. Approximately equal amounts of faeces from each bird were pooled to one sample per isolator. To 2 g of the mixed faeces samples 15 ml broth containing 5000 units penicillin, 50 mg streptomycin and 0.2 µg pimafucin per ml was added, mixed well and centrifuged for 30 minutes at 3000 g. The supernatant was filtered through a 450 nm filter. 0.2 ml aliquots of the undiluted filtrate and of 10^{-1}, 10^{-2} and 10^{-3} dilutions were inoculated into the allantoic cavity of each of five 9 days incubated hatching eggs for virus titration according to Reed and Muench.

Two weeks after challenge blood was collected for HI titration. The challenge was repeated with the residual birds 11 weeks after vaccination. No virus reisolation was attempted but HI determinations were performed 2 weeks after challenge.

RESULTS

HI titres are presented in table 1. It appears that vaccine A produced a more rapid development of circulating antibody than vaccine B when applied in a dose of 500 µl per bird. However, the titre declined more rapidly than after vaccination with emulsion B, resulting in a significantly lower antibody concentration at 9 and 11 weeks post-vaccination (p.v.).

The antibody responses following vaccination with 125 and 62.5 µl doses of vaccine A were low. While some antibody was detected up to 3 weeks p.v., it was practically absent at 9 and 11 weeks p.v.

Birds vaccinated with the oil emulsion based vaccine B produced high concentrations of circulating antibody. The HI titres peaked later than after vaccination with vaccine A but in contrast with the latter, titres remained high up to the end of the experiment. Moreover, even a dose of

62.5 μl of vaccine B still evoked a reasonable antibody response.

TABLE 1   HI titres* after subcutaneous vaccination of five week old SPF chicks with three different doses of two inactivated influenza vaccines and after challenge at 3 and 11 weeks p.v.

	Vaccine						
	A	A	A	B	B	B	None
Dose (μl/bird)	500	125	62.5	500	125	62.5	-
Weeks p.v.							
1	0	0	0	0	0	0	0
2	3	2	1.7	1.3	1	1	1
3	5.3	3	1.6	4.2	2.8	1.3	0
5	3.5	2.4	0.8	5.0	4.0	2.9	0
7	3.3	1.5	0.4	4.7	4.0	3.6	0
9	2.2	0.4	0	4.6	3.2	3.1	0
11	1.9	0.8	0.1	4.5	2.8	2.7	1
2 weeks after challenge							
at week 3 p.v.	3.4	3.2	2.8	4.9	3.9	3.7	5
at week 11 p.v.	5.7	6.9	6.7	4.1	4.1	4.1	6

* Titres are expressed as mean of the logarithms (base 2) of the reciprocal of the highest serum dilutions showing complete HI. Per titration 15 sera were tested. For the number tested after challenge see table 2, "precipitins".

With the exception of the birds vaccinated with 62.5 μl of vaccine A, challenge 3 weeks after vaccination did not result in a rise in antibody titre during the next 2 weeks (compare with titres of 5 week old non-challenged birds). Challenge at 11 weeks p.v. resulted in considerably higher titres 2 weeks later in the birds vaccinated with vaccine A. Only a slight rise of approximately 1.5 log was recorded in birds vaccinated with 125 or 62.5 μl of vaccine B. After challenge of non-vaccinated birds at both ages, the titre increased in the surviving birds to 5 and 6 respectively.

Precipitating antibody had developed only in some birds by 5 weeks after vaccination with 500 μl of vaccine A or with 500 or 125 μl of vaccine B. After challenge at 3 weeks in all vaccinated groups the number of re-actors varied from 1 to 4 out of 15 birds, in contrast to 7 out of 9 surviving birds that had not been vaccinated. By 11 weeks after vaccination no precipitins were detectable. Two weeks after challenge at 11 weeks p.v.

more birds had developed precipitating antibody than after challenge at 3
weeks p.v. (table 2). Especially the birds vaccinated with 500 or 125 µl
of vaccine A or 62.5 µl of vaccine B developed precipitating antibody.

TABLE 2   Morbidity and mortality and precipitating antibodies
           during 2 weeks after challenge 3 and 11 weeks following
           vaccination of SPF chicks with different doses of two
           inactivated influenza vaccines.

| | | | | Vaccine | | | |
	A	A	A	B	B	B	None
Dose (µl/bird)	500	125	62.5	500	125	62.5	-
No. of birds 3 weeks p.v.	15	15	15	15	15	15	15
Sick or/and dead	0	1	2	1	1	2	13
Precipitins*	1/15	4/15	2/12	3/15	1/12	1/14	7/9
No. of birds 11 weeks p.v.	14	15	12	15	15	15	13
Sick or/and dead	4	4	2	0	3	2	11
Precipitins*	9/10	8/11	2/10	6/15	5/14	7/12	2/2

* Number of birds with precipitating antibodies 2 weeks after challenge/
  number of birds examined.

Following challenge at 3 weeks p.v. five of the fifteen non-vaccinated
control birds died whereas another 8 developed serious disease symptoms.
One bird vaccinated with 125 µl and one with 62.5 µl of vaccine B died
whereas some others of each group (see table 2) developed disease symptoms.
Symptoms varied from general rigidness and depression to nervous signs and
some diarrhoea. The combs and wattles of most sick birds became dry and
sometimes black at the tips. Dead birds had laryngitis, tracheitis, congestion of the mucous membranes of the proventriculus and swelling of the
spleen.

Virus was recovered 3 days after challenge from faeces from all groups.
The virus titre varied from 0 (recovery from undiluted faeces) in the non-
vaccinated birds and those vaccinated with 125 µl of vaccine A to 1 in
faeces from birds vaccinated with 125 µl of vaccine B.

After challenge at 11 weeks p.v. 11 out of 13 non-vaccinated birds
died. None out of 15 birds vaccinated with 500 µl of vaccine B showed

disease symptoms. In the groups vaccinated with 125 and 62.5 μl of this vaccine, some mortality and morbidity occurred (table 2).

On the other hand 4 out of 14 birds vaccinated with 500 μl of vaccine A died. Also in the birds vaccinated with 125 and 62.5 μl of this vaccine there was a mortality of 4 out of 15 and 2 out of 12 respectively.

The non-vaccinated birds that died had no circulating antibody at the time of challenge. Equally the majority of the vaccinated birds that became sick or that died had no antibody at that time. However, there were also some birds vaccinated either with vaccine A or B that had HI titres of 3, 4 and 5, that became sick or/and died. On the other hand many birds without antibody (eg 9 out of 15 and 10 out of 12 in the groups vaccinated with 125 and with 62.5 μl of vaccine A respectively) overcame the challenge without developing symptoms.

DISCUSSION

Varying doses of two inactivated vaccines evoked the formation of circulating HI antibody and a varying protection in chicks that had not been exposed before to live virus. Antibody titres increased but also decreased faster after vaccination with vaccine A, an aqueous solution, than with the oil emulsion based vaccine B. Three weeks after vaccination with 500 μl of vaccine A, titres were slightly higher than after vaccination with 500 μl of vaccine B. Although titres of birds vaccinated with 125 and 62.5 μl of vaccine A were not higher than those vaccinated with the same doses of vaccine B, all A vaccinated groups resisted challenge slightly better.

Nine and 11 weeks after vaccination with vaccine A, titres were much lower than after vaccination with vaccine B. Vaccine B gave better protection than vaccine A following challenge at 11 weeks p.v. A greater number of birds injected with 500 and 125 μl of vaccine A than with the same amounts of vaccine B died. There was no difference in morbidity and mortality between the groups vaccinated with 62.5 μl of the vaccines.

The good protection afforded by the 500 and 125 μl doses of vaccine A by 3 weeks and the relatively poor protection by 11 weeks p.v. was reflected in a significant increase in HI titres after challenge of 11 weeks p.v. which was absent or only slight after challenge at 3 weeks p.v. The greater proportions of birds forming precipitins in these groups after challenge at 11 weeks than after challenge at 3 weeks p.v. also indicates a more serious infection.

In the birds vaccinated with 62.5 µl of vaccine A there was no relation between the rise in HI titre and development of precipitins after challenge at 11 weeks p.v.

The lack of a rise in HI titres after challenge at both 3 weeks and 11 weeks after vaccination with 500 and 125 µl of vaccine B indicates a good protection at both ages. In these groups also a smaller proportion of the birds reacted with formation of precipitating antibody compared with the same groups vaccinated with A. However, a large proportion of birds vaccinated with 62.5 µl formed precipitating antibody, indicating a more intensive contact with the challenge virus than in the other two groups.

Both in the vaccinated and in the non-vaccinated birds, virus was re-isolated from faeces samples 3 days after challenge. There were no major differences between virus titres of either vaccinated group, furthermore the titre in the sample from the non-vaccinated birds was not higher than in the samples from vaccinated birds. Provided that the demonstrated virus was newly synthesized, these results indicate that subcutaneous vaccination with inactivated vaccine does not prevent virus shedding via the digestive tract after challenge. More detailed measurements should however be carried out with respect to this aspect of influenza vaccination.

Most birds that died had no circulating antibody at the time of challenge, but some had HI titres of 3, 4 and 5. On the other hand there were many vaccinated birds that resisted challenge (especially in the groups challenged 11 weeks after vaccination with 125 and 62.5 µl of vaccine A), also without antibody or with very low titres. These results indicate that absence of circulating HI antibody in vaccinated birds does not inevitably go together with absence of protection and that the latter is not merely antibody dependent. In contrast, in the majority of the unvaccinated birds, absence of antibody did coincide with a lack of protection.

In general, results indicate that a higher mean antibody titre is associated with a better protection.

REFERENCES

De Jong, W.A. 1978. The influence of the incubation period and the amount of antigen on the haemagglutination inhibition titres to Newcastle disease virus. Tijdschr. Dierg., 103, 104-109.

THE CLASSIFICATION, HOST RANGE AND DISTRIBUTION OF
AVIAN PARAMYXOVIRUSES

D.J. Alexander
Poultry Department
Central Veterinary Laboratory
New Haw, Weybridge, Surrey
KT15 3NB. United Kingdom

I CLASSIFICATION

i)   Paramyxoviruses

Under the present system of classification the virus family
PARAMYXOVIRIDAE is divided into three genera:
Morbillivirus (measles and associated viruses), *Pneumovirus* (respiratory
syncytial virus), *Paramyxovirus*.

The *Paramyxovirus* genus consists of: the mammalian parainfluenza
viruses types 1-5, mumps virus and Newcastle disease virus (NDV) which
is the prototype of the genus. The other avian paramyxoviruses are not
specifically included in the current classification scheme although
clearly possessing all the properties of the paramyxovirus genus and
probably by far outnumbering the paramyxovirus isolates made from
mammals or other animals.

ii)   Avian paramyxovirus nomenclature

The interest in the ecology of avian influenza viruses during the
1970s and the resultant sampling of birds in numerous surveillance
schemes also produced many isolations of paramyxoviruses from avian
species. It became clear, that, since some of these viruses could be
shown to be serologically distinguishable from each other, a system of
nomenclature was necessary if meaningful assessments and comparisons of
the isolates were to be made by different workers.

A pragmatic approach to the problems involved in classification
and nomenclature has resulted in the formation of a practicable system
in which paramyxoviruses isolated from birds have been effectively
regarded as a subgenus of the paramyxovirus genus. Further, the avian
paramyxoviruses have been placed, on the basis of serological tests,
into distinct groups. Currently there are nine recognised serogroups
termed PMV-1 to PMV-9, adopting the nomenclature recommended by Tumova
et al (1979a). In addition, general usage has resulted in the adoption

of isolate designation using the system recommended by the WHO Expert
Committee (1980) for influenza isolates. This means that an isolate
name includes 1. serotype 2. species or type of bird from which it was
isolated 3. geographical location of isolation – country or state 4.
reference number or reference name, if any 5. year of isolation. eg.
PMV-1/pigeon/England/561/83, PMV-8/pintail/Wakuya/20/78, PMV-3/turkey/
England/MPH/81.

The first isolate of each group or designated isolates have been
proposed as prototype strains for each of the serogroups. These are
listed in Table 1.

TABLE 1   Avian paramyxovirus isolates regarded
             prototype strains.

PMV-1	Newcastle disease virus
PMV-2	chicken/California/Yucaipa/56
PMV-3	*i) turkey/Wisconsin/68
	*ii) parakeet/Netherlands/449/75
PMV-4	duck/Hong Kong/D3/75
PMV-5	budgerigar/Japan/Kunitachi/75
PMV-6	duck/Hong/Kong/199/77
PMV-7	dove/Tennessee/4/75
PMV-8	goose/Delaware/1053/76
PMV-9	duck/New York/22/78

Viruses under investigation as putative new serotypes:

PMV-?	avian faeces/England/B114/80
PMV-?	goose/England/77/83

* see text.

iii) Serotypes

No attempt has been made to produce a definition of a serotype
for the avian paramyxoviruses. Initially differentiation into serogroups
was based on serological tests such as the haemagglutination inhibition
(HI) test, but, in more recent years, other tests and virus properties
have been used.

Using HI tests several authors have reported minor crosss reaction
between PMV-1 and PMV-4 serotypes (Kessler et al, 1979); PMV-1 and PMV-
8, PMV-1 and PMV-9, PMV-3 and PMV-8, PMV-3 and PMV-9, PMV-4 and PMV-8

(Alexander *et al*, 1983b); PMV-7? and PMV-1, PMV-7 and PMV-3 (Gough and Alexander, 1983); PMV-2 and PMV-6 (Shortridge *et al*, 1980). The degree of relationship has varied enormously from one report to another and in some instances may be related to the use of mammalian antisera. However the most frequently reported cross-relationship between PMV-3 and PMV-1 appears to represent close antigenic relationships between these two groups of viruses and Alexander *et al* (1979) were able to show that chickens could be protected, to some extent, from challenge with virulent NDV if previously infected with some PMV-3 viruses. Surviving birds showed increase in both NDV and PMV-3 HI titres. Similarly in NDV-vaccinated turkeys naturally infected with PMV-3 viruses NDV HI titres were boosted in direct correlation to the PMV-3 HI titres obtained (Alexander *et al*, 1983a).

Neuraminidase inhibition tests have also been used to type avian paramyxoviruses and these have tended to give similar results to the HI tests (Kessler *et al*, 1979, Nerome *et al*, 1984, Tumova *et al*, 1984).

Kida and Yanagawa (1981) isolated the HN and M polypeptides of representative avian paramyxoviruses to use in immunodouble diffusion (IDD) tests. They examined 18 isolates which formed six groups, using either polypeptide, each of which corresponded to a serotype defined by HI and other serological tests. One important observation was that in IDD tests no low level relationships between serotypes similar to those seen in HI tests were observed. Abenes *et al* (1983) compared the HN and M polypeptides of PMV-7/dove/Tn/4/75 and PMV-7?/pigeon/Otaru/76 in IDD tests. They concluded that these viruses had related HN polypeptides, which accounted for their relationship in HI tests, but distinct M polypeptides. These authors considered that the two viruses should be placed in separate groups in accord with the suggestion by Kida and Yanagawa (1981) that IDD tests with the M polypeptide should be used to type avian paramyxoviruses. However in view of the detected antigenic relationships between dove/TN/4/75 and pigeon/Otaru/76 separation would appear premature until further analysis of additional related viruses has been done.

Alexander *et al* (1983b) used IDD tests with whole disrupted viruses and chicken antisera to demonstrate the distinctiveness of subtypes PMV-8 and PMV-9 and the similarity of different isolates, from Japan and USA, falling within the PMV-8 group.

In a novel approach to avian paramyxovirus typing Ishida *et al* (1985) prepared guinea pig antisera to the isolated HN polypeptides of viruses representing PMV-1 to PMV-7. They confirmed the groupings obtained in studies using sera prepared against whole virus by HI, neuraminidase inhibition and IDD tests.

Techniques which do not employ a serological reaction have also been used to group avian paramyxoviruses.

Alexander and Collins (1981) used polyacrylamide gel electrophoresis for analysis of the structural polypeptides of 23 avian paramyxoviruses. They showed that the viruses tested could be placed into groups, which correspond to the five serotypes studied, on the basis of the similarity of the polypeptide profiles. However they reported considerable variation within the serogroups. In subsequent studies polypeptide profiles have been used to confirm the serological findings and support the similarities or distinctiveness of new isolates.

Analyses of the RNA genomes by T1 oligonucleotide mapping indicated that serologically related viruses produce basically similar maps. However the finer variations and similarities detected related to the origins of the isolated viruses (Nerome *et al*, 1983, 1984).

The overall trend of the use of sophisticated techniques has been to confirm the avian paramyxovirus groupings made on the basis of simple HI tests. However in one study there has been some evidence of relationships between two of the serotypes considered to be quite distinct. Hoshi *et al* (1983) prepared monoclonal antibodies against the HN polypetide of Taka virus, a PMV-1 variant, and one of these antibodies gave an HI titre with the homologous virus and two PMV-2 viruses that were tested.

iv) Variations within serotypes

A further important consideration in the classification of avian paramyxoviruses is the degree of variation that occurs within a serogroup. This is especially important when relatively few isolates are available as it is difficult to know, using limited techniques, whether or not detectable heterology between two viruses represents different serotypes or merely extremes of a spectrum of antigenic variation.

Little or no variation has been reported in serological tests using viruses of serotypes PMV-4, PMV-5, PMV-6, PMV-8 or PMV-9 although

more stringent tests such as polypeptide analysis (Alexander and
Collins, 1981, Alexander *et al*, 1983b) or oligonucleotide mapping of
the genome (Nerome *et al*,1983, 1984) have indicated some variation
within these serotypes.

PMV-1 viruses are usually regarded as a homologous group and the
strategy behind NDV vaccination of commercial poultry is based on this
assumption. However some serological tests have revealed minor variations between strains apparently identical in HI tests and occasionally
viruses exhibiting marked variation even in HI tests have been isolated
(Arias-Ibarrondo *et al*, 1978; Hannoun, 1977; Alexander *et al*, 1984a).

Several groups have prepared monoclonal antibodies to PMV-1
strains (Russell and Alexander, 1983, Nishikawa *et al*, 1983; Iorio *et
al*, 1984; Ishida *et al*, 1985) and have used these to demonstrate differences between PMV-1 isolates. Russell and Alexander (1983) and Alexander
et al (1984a) were able to place NDV isolates into nine distinct groups
on the basis of the ability of the viruses to induce binding of the
monoclonal antibodies to infected MDBK cells. Viruses placed in the
same group tended to share biological and epidemiological properites.

Other workers have distinguished between PMV-1 strains by Oligonucleotide mapping (McMillan and Hanson, 1982) and one dimensional
polypeptide mapping (Nagy and Lomniczi, 1984).

PMV-2 viruses have shown wide variation in serological tests
including HI tests (Alexander, 1980) frequently two widely diverging
viruses both showing close homology with a third. Other isolates have
shown asymmetrical cross relationships. Some variation has also been
reported in the structural polypeptide profiles of PMV-2 isolates
(Alexander and Collins, 1981). To date none of the variations between
isolates of PMV-2 viruses have been related to epidemiological or
biological properties.

Variations also exist between PMV-3 viruses. In general terms
serological tests have indicated PMV-3 viruses isolated from either
turkeys or psittacines have shown closer relationships with viruses from
the same source (Alexander *et al*, 1982). Alexander and Collins (1984)
showed that polypeptide profiles of the structural polypeptides of
PMV-3 turkey isolates from Great Britain had much closer identity to
isolates from turkeys in the USA than they did to psittacine PMV-3
isolates.

v)   Relationship to mammalian paramyxoviruses

Investigations into the possible relationships between avian and mammalian paramyxoviruses have generally been very limited and restricted to screening new isolates in HI or other serological tests. Usually such testing has proved negative (Alexander, 1980) and is in keeping with the marked differences in growth, structural and biological properties between the mammalian and most avian paramyxoviruses. However, some studies have reported some relationships between PMV-1 and mumps (Chanock and Coates, 1964); PMV-2 and parainfluenza 2 (Dinter et al, 1964); PMV-2 and parainfluenza 3 (Starke et al, 1977); PMV-1, PMV-3 and mumps (Tumova et al, 1979), PMV-1 and parainfluenza 1 (Brostrom et al, 1971).

In a more recent study Tumova et al (1984) showed a relationship between PMV-4 viruses and mumps virus by HI, complement fixation and IDD tests.

The relationships reported between mammalian and avian paramyxoviruses tend to be, to some extent, conflicting and confusing. It is clear that before firm conclusions can be drawn further work is required, not least to exclude the possibility of non-specific cross-reactivity in closely controlled tests.

II   HOST RANGE AND DISTRIBUTION

In natural infections individual serotypes of avian paramyxoviruses tend to show a marked demarcation for specific groups or types of birds. However experimental or artificial infections would indicate that most of the avian paramyxoviruses are able to infect a wide variety of avian species; so that affinities for any group of birds may be more a result of lack of intermingling of different groups rather that any particular host specificity or "species barrier".

Data on the presence of avian paramyxovirus infection of different species of bird depend very much on whether or not any given bird has been held captive and sampled. Birds that fall into this category may come from three sources: i) trapped or hunter-killed wild birds specifically sampled for viruses ii) captive caged birds, which may be routinely sampled at time of export or import or during quarantine periods iii) domestic poultry. Reported paramyxovirus isolations for these three groups are summarized in Tables 2-4 and will be dealt with separately.

TABLE 2   Isolation of avian paramyxoviruses from feral birds.

Type of bird order or family	Avian paramyxovirus sub-type	Country reporting isolation
Passeriformes (perching birds)	PMV-2	German Democratic Republic Senegal, Indonesia, Kenya, Czechoslovakia, Israel, Japan, India
Anatidae* (ducks and geese)	PMV-2	Israel
	PMV-4	USA, Czechoslovakia, Japan Federal Republic of Germany, Great Britain, New Zealand,
	PMV-6	Canada, FRG, Japan, Czechoslovakia.
	PMV-8	USA, Japan
Columbidae (doves and pigeons)	PMV7**	USA, Japan, Great Britain
Rallidae (coots)	PMV-2	Israel
	PMV-4	Czechoslovakia, FRG.
Ardeidae (cattle egret)	PMV-2	Israel
Spheniscidae (penguins)	unclassified	Antartica

* Two unclassified paramyxoviruses isolated from waterfowl faeces and
  a goose in Geat Britain may represent further subtypes.
**Includes isolates from doves provisionally placed in the PMV-7 group.

i)   Feral birds

In most cases paramyxoviruses have been isolated from trapped or
hunter-killed wild birds showing no signs of disease. Generally surveillance of such birds had not been primarily aimed at avian paramyxoviruses but has, more usually, been concerned with the ecology of
influenza viruses. In this context such surveillance programmes yielding avian paramyxoviruses may have been restricted to groups of birds
known to be carriers of influenza viruses, such as waterfowl. This may
affect the usefulness of making generalizations concerning the predomi-

nant groups of birds infected with avian paramyxoviruses based on the currently available data. Notwithstanding the possible uncertainty, some assessment of birds in which the different types of paramyxovirus are naturally endemic can be made.

Isolates of PMV-6 viruses made in Canada (Hinshaw personal communication), Federal Republic of Germany (Ottis and Bachmann, 1983) Japan (Abenes *et al*, 1982; Mikami *et al*, 1982) and Czechoslovakia (Tumova *et al*, 1984) were all isolated from ducks.

Isolates of PMV-8 have been obtained only from waterfowl, Canada geese *(Branta canadensis)* in the USA and pintail ducks *(Anas acuta)* in Japan (Alexander *et al*, 1983b).

PMV-4 viruses have also been isolated predominantly from feral birds of the order Anseriformes but there have also been reports of isolates from coots *(Fulica atra)* and from a wild pheasant (Ottis and Bachmann, 1983; Tumova *et al*, 1984).

PMV-7 viruses and those placed provisionally in the group have only been isolated from members of the Columbiformes order (Gough and Alexander, 1983; Alexander, unpublished).

PMV-2 viruses would appear to be endemic in birds of the order Passeriformes in many parts of the world (Table 2). However there have been reports of isolation of PMV-2 viruses from trapped psittacines in Indonesia (Ksiazek, 1980 personal communication) but this may have been a result of infection after trapping due to contact with passerines. In Israel PMV-2 viruses have also been isolated from mallards *(Anas platyrhyncos)*, cattle egrets *(Ardeola (Bubulcus?)ibis)* and coots *(Fulica atra)* during a widespread epizootic in turkeys (Lipkind *et al*, 1982a, 1982b).

There have been no reports of isolations of PMV-3, PMV-5 or PMV-9 viruses from feral birds.

ii) Captive caged birds

The vast majority of caged birds are from two orders: Passeriformes and Psittaciformes and it would be expected that isolation of avian paramyxoviruses from such birds would reflect the presence of these viruses in the feral populations.

TABLE 3   Isolations of avian paramyxoviruses from captive caged birds

Bird order	Avian paramyxovirus sub-type	Country reporting isolation
Psittaciformes	PMV-2	Japan, Great Britain, USA Indonesia
	PMV-3	Great Britain, USA, Netherlands, Federal Republic of Germany, Japan
	PMV-5	Japan
Passeriformes	PMV-2	Japan, N.Ireland, Great Britain, USA, Indonesia, Senegal
	PMV-3	USA, Great Britain, Japan, Federal Republic of Germany

In Great Britain virus isolation is attempted from birds dying in quarantine and between 1976-1984 119 avian paramyxoviruses, other than PMV-1, were isolated from identified birds from this source. Seventy-four viruses were identified as of PMV-2 serotype, 67 (91%) of these were isolated from passerine birds and 7 (9%) from psittacines. Another 43 viruses were of PMV-3 serotype, 8 (19%) from passerines and 35 (81%) from psittacines (Alexander, unpublished). Much larger numbers were isolated from identified birds in quarantine in the USA during 1974-1981 (Senne et al, 1983) but basically similar proportions were obtained. Of 665 PMV-2 isolates 580 (87%) were from passerines and 85 (13%) were from psittacines. While for PMV-3 isolates, from a total of 433, 46 (11%) were from passerines and 387 (89%) from psittacines.

The isolations from birds in quarantine indicate that PMV-2 viruses primarily infect passerines and PMV-3 viruses primarily infect psittacines but that birds from either order may be infected by the other virus when in contact with infected birds.

The frequent isolation of PMV-3 viruses from psittacines in quarantine compared to the absence of isolations from feral birds, probably reflects the sparcity of studies in feral psittacines, particularly in

geographical areas where the virus is endemic, rather than the perpetu-
ation of the virus in quarantine or transit premises. However, investigations into the origins of caged birds rarely reach satisfactory
conclusions due to practices of exporting via intermediate holding
countries or mixing of birds, even from different continents and hemis-
pheres during transit.

PMV-5 isolates were related to a unique epizootic which occurred
in pet budgerigars *(Melopsittacus undulatus)* in Japan during 1974-1976
(Nerome *et al*, 1978), there was no evidence of natural spread to birds
of any other species.

iii) Domestic poultry

Isolations of PMV-4 and PMV-6 viruses from commercial ducks and
geese in Hong Kong (Shortridge & Alexander, 1978: Shortridge *et al*,
1980) were presumably a result of infection due to direct contact with
feral waterfowl occurring during the rearing of birds on open ponds.
Turek *et al* (1984) using sentinel commercial ducks, placed in the
vicinity of wild aquatic birds, showed that transfer of PMV-4 viruses
will take place.

Small passerines are frequent visitors to and invaders of poultry
houses and this would suggest a method by which PMV-2 viruses could be
introduced to domestic poultry. Lipkind *et al* (1982a) suggested that
the introduction of PMV-2 viruses responsible for the epizootic in turkeys in 1979 may have been by migratory birds. However Lang *et al*
(1975), after investigations of PMV-2 outbreak on three separate turkey
farms in Canada, stressed that each of the farms had close trading
links with California, USA where PMV-2 viruses were known to be present in turkeys. They further speculated that the Canadian outbreaks
were the result of three separate introductions from California. This
stresses the possible importance in domestic poultry trade in the desem-
mination of PMV-2, and other avian paramyxoviruses.

PMV-3 infections of domestic poultry offer even stronger evidence
that introduction into different areas and countries occurs as a result
of contact with infected domestic poultry rather than by repeated introduction by feral birds as there have been no isolations of PMV-3 viruses
from feral birds. In addition, Alexander and Collins (1984) used polyacrylamide gel electrophoresis analysis of the structural polypeptides

TABLE 4 Isolations of avian paramyxoviruses from domestic poultry

Type of Bird	Avian paramyxovirus sub-type	Country reporting isolates	Associated disease
Fowl	PMV-2	USA, USSR, Japan, Israel, India	Mild respiratory disease and egg production problems. If complicated due to other organisms exacerbation may occur with resulting high mortality.
	PMV-4	Hong Kong	none
Turkeys	PMV-2	USA, Canada. Italy, Israel, France	Similar to disease in chickens but generally more severe.
	PMV-3	USA, Canada, England, France	Similar to PMV-2 infections but generally manifested as marked egg production drops.
	PMV-6	Canada	Mild respiratory disease and egg production problems
Ducks & Geese	PMV-4	Hong Kong Czechoslovakia	none
	PMV-6	Hong Kong	none
	PMV-9	USA	none

of different PMV-3 viruses to show that islolates from turkeys in Great Britain and USA were similar but were distinguishable from psittacine PMV-3 isolates.

III COMMENT

A period of nearly 30 years separated the isolation and identification of the first avian paramyxovirus, PMV-1 (Doyle, 1927), in 1927 and the second, PMV-2 (Bankowski *et al,* 1960) in 1956. Viruses of the third serotype, PMV-3, were not recognised until 1967 (Tumova *et al,* 1979b). However between 1975-1978 isolations of viruses forming a further six serotypes, PMV-4 to PMV-9, were made, which represents the great increase in interest in avian paramyxoviruses and wild birds as virus carriers which occurred at that time.

As more isolations of paramyxoviruses have been made from birds the majority have been placed in the recognised serotypes. However several viruses are currently under investigation as representing distinct serogroups and it seems inevitable that further serotypes will be identified. In addition to the recognition of new serotypes considerable antigenic diversity has been seen within the existing serogroups. Although the autonomy of the recognised serotypes has been supported by most antigenic tests there is some evidence of cross-relationships between different types which may represent phylogenic relationships. Such variations within the avian paramyxoviruses may eventually necessitate the formation of subgroups or supergroups.

Representatives of the majority of the avian paramyxovirus serotypes have been isolated from wild birds and there is some evidence of specific relationships between certain viruses and the type of bird in which they may be endemic. The presence of paramyxoviruses in feral birds, particularly small birds such as passerines which frequently invade poultry houses, indicates a ready source for spread to domestic poultry. There is also good evidence to show that like NDV (PMV-1) other avian paramyxoviruses may circulate amongst domestic poultry causing economic loss and disease problems which may be exacerbated by the presence of other organisms.

REFERENCES

Abenes, G.B., Okazaki, K., Fukushi, H., Kida, H., Honda, E., Yagyu, K., Tsuji, M., Sato, H., Ono, E., Yanagawa, R. and Yamauchi, N. 1982. Isolation of ortho- and paramyxoviruses from feral birds in Hokkaido, Japan - 1980 and 1981. Jpn. J. Vet. Sci., 10, 703-708.

Abenes, G.B., Kida, H. and Yanagawa, R. 1983. Avian paramyxoviruses possessing antigenically related HN but distinct M proteins. Archiv. Virol. 77 71-76

Alexander, D.J. (1980). Avian paramyxovirus. Vet.Bull., 50, 737-752.

Alexander, D.J. and Collins, M.S. (1981). The structural polypeptides of avian paramyxoviruses. Archiv. Virol. 67, 309-323.

Alexander, D.J., Chettle, N.J. and Parsons, G. 1979a. Resistance of chickens to challenge with the virulent Herts 33 strain of Newcastle disease virus induced by prior infection with serologically distinct avian paramyxoviruses. Res.Vet.Sci., 26, 198-201.

Alexander, D.J., Allan, W.H., Parsons, G. and Collins, M.S. 1982. Identification of paramyxoviruses isolated from birds dying in quarantine in Great Britain during 1980 to 1981. Vet.Rec., 111, 571-574.

Alexander, D.J., Pattison, M. and Macpherson, I. 1983a. Avian paramyxoviruses of PMV-3 serotype in British turkeys. Avian Path., 12, 469-482.

Alexander, D.J., Hinshaw, V.S., Collins, M.S. and Yamane, N. 1983b. Characterization of viruses which represent further distinct serotypes (PMV-8 and PMV-9) of avian paramyxoviruses. Archiv. Virol., 78, 29-36.

Alexander, D.J., Russell, P.H. and Collins, M.S. 1984. Paramyxovirus type 1 infections of racing pigeons: 1 characterization of isolated viruses. Vet. Rec., 114, 444-446.

Arias-Ibarrondo, J., Mikami, T., Yamamoto, H., Furuta, Y., Ishioka, S., Okada, K. and Sato, G. 1978. Studies on a paramyxovirus isolated from Japanese sparrow-hawks (Accipter virgatus gularis). Jap. J. Vet.Sci., 40, 315-323.

Bankowski, R.A., Corstvet, R.E. and Clark, G.T. 1960. Isolation of an unidentified agent from the respiratory tract of chickens. Science., 132, 292-293

Brostrom, M.A., Bruening, G. and Bankowski, R.A. 1971. Comparisons of neuraminidases of paramyxoviruses with immunologically dissimilar haemagglutinins. Virology., 46, 856-865.

Chanock, R.M. and Coates, H.V. 1964. Myxoviruses - a comparative description. In. "Newcastle Disease: an evolving pathogen" (Ed. by R.P. Hanson) (Univ. Wisconsin Press: Madison). pp. 279-198.

Dinter, Z., Hermondsson, S. and Hermondsson, L. 1964. Studies on myxovirus Yucaipa; its classification as a member of the paramyxovirus group. Virology., 22, 297-304.

Doyle, T.M. 1927. A hitherto unrecorded disease of fowls due to a filter-passing virus. J. Comp. Path. Therap., 40, 144-169.

Gough, R.E. and Alexander, D.J. 1983. The isolation and preliminary characterisation of a paramyxovirus from collared doves (Streptapelia decaocto). Avian Path., 12, 125-134.

Hannoun, C. 1977. Isolation from birds of viruses with human neuraminidases. Devs. Biol. Standard. 39, 469-472.

Hoshi, S., Mikami, T., Nagata, K., Onuma, M. and Izawa, H. 1983. Monoclonal antibodies against a paramyxovirus isolated from a Japanese sparrow-hawk *(Accipter virugatus gularis)*. Archiv. Virol., 76, 145-151.

Ishida, M., Nerome, K., Matsumoto, M., Mikami, T. and Oya, A. 1985 Characterization of reference strains of Newcastle disease virus (NDV) and NDV-like isolates by monoclonal antibodies to HN subunits. (In press).

Kessler, N., Aymard, M. and Calvet, A. 1979. A study of a new strain of paramyxoviruses isolated from wild ducks: antigenic and biological properties. J. gen. Virol., 43, 273-282.

Kida, H. and Yanagawa, R. 1981. Classification of avian paramyxoviruses by immunodiffusion on the basis of antigenic specificity of their M protein antigens. J. gen. Virol., 52, 103-111.

Lang, G., Gagnon, A. and Howell, J. 1975. Occurrence of paramyxoviruses Yucaipa in Canadian poultry. Canad. Vet. J., 16, 233-237.

Lipkind, M.A., Shihmanter, E., Weisman, Y., Aronovici, A. and Shoham, D. 1982a. Characterization of Yucaipa - like avian paramyxoviruses isolated in Israel from domestic and wild birds. Ann. Virol., 133E, 157-161.

Lipkind, M.A., Weisman, Y., Shihmanter, E. and Aronovici, A. 1982b. Isolation of Yucaipa-like avian paramyxoviruses from migrating coots *(Fulica atra)* wintering in Israel. Zbl. Bact. Hyg. I. Abt. Orig. A253 159-163.

McMillan, B.C. and Hanson R.P. 1982. Differentiation of exotic strains of Newcastle disease virus by oligonucleotide fingerprinting. Avian Dis., 26, 332-339.

Mikami, T., Izawa, H., Kodama, H., Onuma, M., Sato, A., Kobayashi, S., Ishida, M. and Nerome, K. 1982. Isolation of ortho- and paramyxoviruses from migrating feral ducks in Hokkaido. Archiv. Virol., 74, 211-217.

Nagy, E. and Lomniczi, B. 1984. Differentiation of Newcastle disease virus strains by one-dimensional peptide mapping. J. Virol. Meths., 9, 227-235.

Nerome, K., Nakayama, M., Ishida, M., Fukumi, H. and Morita, A. 1978. Isolation of a new avian paramyxovirus from budgerigar *(Melopsittacus undulatus)*. J. gen. Virol., 38, 293-301.

Nerome, K., Ishida, M., Oya, A. and Bosshard, S. 1983. Genomic analysis of antigenically related avian paramyxoviruses. J. gen. Virol., 64, 465-470.

Nerome, K., Shibata, M., Kobayashi, S., Yamaguchi, R., Yoshioka, Y., Isida, M. and Oya. A. 1984. Immunological and genomic analysis of two serotypes of avian paramyxovirus isolated from wild ducks in Japan. J. Virol., 50, 649-653.

Nishikawa, K., Isomura, S., Suzuki, S. Watanabe, E., Hamaguchi, M., Yoshida, T. and and Nagai, Y. 1983. Monoclonal antibodies to the HN glycoprotein of Newcastle disease virus. Biological characterization and use for strain comparisons. Virology., 130, 318-330.

Ottis, K. and Bachmann, P.A. 1983. Isolations and characterization of ortho- and paramyxoviruses from feral birds in Europe. Zbl. Vet. Med. B., 30, 22-35..

Senne, D.A., Pearson, J.E., Miller, L.D. and Gustafson, G.A. 1983. Virus isolations from pet birds submitted from importation into the United States. Avian Dis., 27, 731-744.

Shortridge, K.F. and Alexander, D.J. 1978. Incidence and preliminary
    characterisation of a hitherto unreported, serologically distinct
    avian paramyxovirus isolated in Hong Kong. Res. Vet. Sci., 25,
    128–130.
Shortridge, K.F., Alexander, D.J. and Collins, M.S. 1980. Isolation
    and properties of viruses from poultry in Hong Kong which repre-
    sents a new (sixth) distinct group of avian paramyxoviruses.
    J. gen. Virol., 49, 255–262.
Starke, G., Alexander, D.J., Nymadawa, P. and Konstantinow-Siebelist, I.
    1977. Serological relationships between certain avian and animal
    paramyxoviruses. Acta Virol., 21, 503–506.
Tumova, B., Stumpa, A., Janout, V., Uvizl, M. and Chmela, J. 1979a.
    A further member of the Yucaipa group isolated from the common
    wren (Troglodytes troglodytes). Acta. Virol., 23, 504–507.
Tumova, B., Robinson J.H. and Easterday, B.C. 1979b. A hitherto
    unreported paramyxovirus of turkeys. Res. Vet. Sci., 27, 135–140.
Tumova, B., Turek, R., Kubinova, I., Stumpa, A. and Ciampor, F. 1984.
    Incidence of paramyxoviruses in free-living birds in 1978-1982.
    Acta Virol., 28, 114–121.
Turek, R., Gresikova, M. and Tumova, B. 1984. Isolation of influenza A
    virus and paramyxoviruses from sentinel domestic ducks. Acta
    Virol., 28, 156–158.
WHO Expert Committee. 1980. A revision of the system of nomenclature
    for influenza viruses: a WHO memorandum. Bull. Wld. Hlth. Org.,
    58, 585–591

PARAMYXOVIRUS TYPE 1 INFECTION IN PIGEONS

H. Vindevogel, J.-P. Duchatel

Clinic of Avian Diseases
Faculty of Veterinary Medicine
University of Liège
45 rue des Vétérinaires
B-1070 Brussels, Belgium

INTRODUCTION

Newcastle disease (ND) is a severe disease of poultry but other species of birds can be infected including domestic pigeons and doves (Vindevogel et al., 1972; Mousa et al., 1982; Sabban et al., 1982).

Usually, ND has occurred in pigeons during widespread epizootics of ND in domestic poultry and pigeons have been infected as a result of contact with diseased domestic poultry (Vindevogel et al., 1972).

In 1980, several lentogenic classical NDV strains were isolated from pigeons with respiratory disease and serological investigations performed at the same period showed that 7% of racing pigeons in Belgium and 19% in France possessed specific antibodies (Vindevogel, 1981; Vindevogel et al., 1982b; Landré et al., 1982).

In 1981, clinical signs resembling the neurotropic form of ND began to occur in the racing pigeon population of the Mediterranean countries (Vindevogel et al., 1982a) and a virus isolated from Italian diseased pigeons was characterised as a mesogenic Paramyxovirus type 1 (PMV 1) strain (Vindevogel et al., 1983). In 1983, the infection spread throughout continental Europe and Great Britain (Alexander et al., 1984).

CLASSICAL NDV INFECTION IN PIGEONS

1. Epizootiology.

Pigeons can be infected by NDV velogenic strains during the epizootic periods and by lentogenic strains in between (Vindevogel et al., 1972, 1982b). Pigeons therefore participate in the natural transmission of the infection.

Infection is transmitted through direct and indirect contact with nasal secretions and faeces. The incubation period varies from 6 to 16 days (Vindevogel et al., 1972).

2. Disease signs, pathology.

68

a. Velogenic NDV infection:

After infection with a velogenic strain of NDV, respiratory, digestive and nervous symptoms appear in the dove-cot. Pigeons show conjunctivitis, rhinitis, dyspnoea and congestion of pharyngeal and laryngeal mucous membranes. These symptoms are accompanied by watery or haemorrhagic diarrhoea. Nervous signs consist of tremors of the neck and the wings, torticollis, paralysis, problems in equilibrium and vision and inco-ordinated movements (Vindevogel et al., 1972).

The morbidity percentage reaches 70% and that of mortality 40% (Vindevogel et al., 1972).

The virus is eliminated in the faeces during the acute phase of the disease but not during convalescence. The virus may persist in the lungs and in the trachea as long as 4 weeks post-inoculation and in the brain until the end of the 5th week. The period of viral excretion by pigeons is therefore relatively short and recovered birds do not become asymptomatic carriers (Vindevogel et al., 1972).

b. Lentogenic NDV infection:

After inoculation with lentogenic strains, pigeons show only mild respiratory symptoms 6 days later and sometimes conjunctivitis (Vindevogel, 1981; Vindevogel et al., 1982b). The virus can be isolated from the pharynx from day 3 to day 7 post infection (Vindevogel, 1981; Vindevogel et al., 1982b).

PMV 1 INFECTION OF PIGEONS

1. Properties of the "pigeon" PMV 1.

a. Antigenic properties:

The virus was first isolated in 1981 from Italian pigeons and characterised as a PMV 1 strain (Vindevogel et al., 1982a, 1983). After dissemination of the infection in Europe in 1983, Alexander et al. (1984) confirmed the classification of the "pigeon" strains within the type 1 serotype of avian paramyxoviruses. However, the "pigeon" viruses can be distinguished from more classical PMV 1 viruses by the significantly different titres obtained in haemagglutination inhibition tests (HI tests), particularly when pigeon antisera are used instead of conventional chicken antisera (Duchatel et al., 1985a), by the failure of mouse monoclonal antibodies directed against the HN1 epitope of NDV Ulster 2 C strain to inhibit their haemagglutinating activity and a unique binding pattern seen with the nine mouse monoclonal antibodies (Alexander et al., 1984).

b. Biological properties:

The first strain of "pigeon" PMV 1 isolated from Italian pigeons in 1981 and Belgian strains isolated in 1983 and 84 were shown to possess the biological properties of mesogenic strains (table 1) and thus display some virulence for chickens.

TABLE 1   Pathogenicity index of "pigeon" PMV 1 strains

Strains	ICPI	IVPI
strain 135/81*	for chicken 1.25 for pigeon 0.51	for chicken 0.49 for pigeon 0.50
strain D/83**	for chicken 1.40	for chicken 0.51
strains 1984 (1)***	for chicken 1.50	for chicken 0.75
(2)	1.40	0.45
(3)	1.10	0.30

  * Vindevogel et al., 1982a;   ** Viaene et al., 1983;
*** personal results.

Guittet and Bennejean (1984) and Heil (1984) also characterised the majority of the "pigeon" strains isolated in France and in Germany as mesogenic. Strains are principally neurotropic and viscerotropic (Duchatel et al., 1985a).

2. Epizootiology.

a. Distribution of the infection:

"Pigeon" PMV 1 strains have to date been isolated in Mediterranean countries, Germany, Belgium, Netherlands, France, Great Britain, Austria and Israel (Vindevogel et al., 1982a; Richter et al.; 1983; Viaene et al., 1983, Guittet and Bennejean, 1984; Alexander et al., 1984; Schusser et al., 1984; Weisman et al., 1984; Lumeji and Stam, 1985). Infection has also reached Japan and the USA (Nunomura, 1984; Chalmers, 1985).

b. Transmission of the infection:

In the experimental disease, the incubation period varies from 4 to 18 days (Duchatel et al., 1985). In field outbreaks, new clinical cases may appear in an infected dove-cot up to 5 weeks after the onset of the disease.

Infected pigeons excrete virus in the laryngeal secretions from the second to the 9th day after infection and in the faeces from the second to the 14th day (Figure 1). Infection can thus be transmitted through direct and indirect contact with nasal secretions and faeces even during the incubation period. Pigeon breeders play an important role in the disease transmission during handling as well as at race meetings.

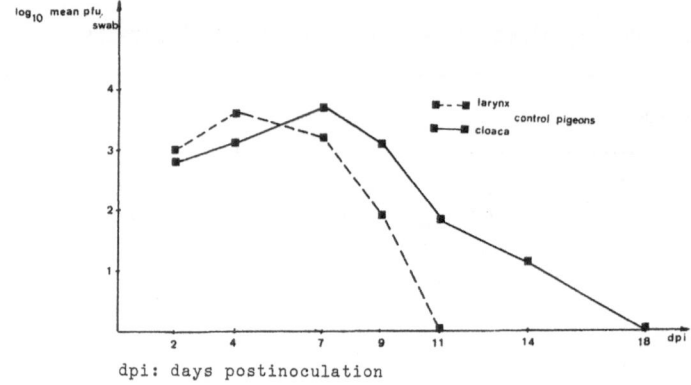

dpi: days postinoculation

Fig. 1   Means of numbers of viral particles isolated in swabs of larynx and cloaca of pigeons inoculated with a "pigeon" PMV 1 strain (From Duchatel et al., 1985a).

3. Disease signs, pathology.

"Pigeon" PMV 1 disease resembles the neurotropic form of ND. Nervous symptoms are accompanied or preceded by watery or haemorrhagic diarrhoea. Diseased pigeons will consequently drink enormously. Respiratory symptoms are not a feature.

Atypical signs may be observed in some infected dove-cots as persistent diarrhoea without the appearance of nervous symptoms.

If pigeons become infected during the moult, remiges or coverts may be badly grown; fragile rachis, poorly developed barbes and barbules and broken feathers may be observed.

At necropsy, few lesions are visible except for catarrhal or haemorrhagic enteritis during the acute phase of the infection.

Morbidity varies from 30 to 70% but mortality does not exceed 10% if uncomplicated by secondary bacterial or parasitic infections. In such cases, mortality can be over 30%.

4. Prognosis.

Diseased valuable racing pigeons can be saved. Indeed, many pigeons, even those showing severe nervous troubles, can recover entirely after a convalescence of 2 to 6 months and their orientation sense will not be damaged. But diarrhoea may persist as long as several months, in which case the flying performance of the bird will of course be diminished.

PROPHYLAXIS AND CONTROL

Studies by Erickson et al. (1980) and Vindevogel et al. (1981, 1982b) reported that LaSota strain may be a good candidate for vaccinating pigeons against ND infection. Indeed, pigeons vaccinated intraocularly and intra-nasally showed a weak seroconversion but were protected during 2 months against a challenge with a velogenic strain of NDV and were able to reduce its level of excretion.

However, as lentogenic NDV strains display some virulence for pigeons and are excreted 3 to 7 days after inoculation, inactivated vaccines are preferable for vaccinating racing pigeons (Vindevogel, 1981; Vindevogel et al., 1982b).

Inactivated oil emulsion vaccines are not well tolerated by racing pigeons. After one injection, one pigeon in 10 000 may die of shock. Two per cent of birds may develop a granuloma at the site of injection. Vac-cination may reactivate herpesvirus (Pigeon herpesvirus 1), of which the majority of pigeons are latent carriers, and one per cent of birds may consequently persent 2 to 3 weeks after vaccination with severe conjunct-ivitis or sinusitis (Vindevogel and Duchatel, 1985).

For these reasons, Vindevogel et al. (1984) and Duchatel et al. (1985a) have developed an inactivated aqueous vaccine for racing pigeons.

The vaccine contains purified inactivated LaSota strain suspended in an aqueous adjuvant (PD solution, Duphar B.V.*) (10^9 EID_{50} before in-activation/0.2 ml; 0.2 ml pro dose 1).

Subcutaneous injection of the vaccine does not provoke any secondary reaction (Duchatel et al., 1985a).

In vaccination trials, antibodies were detectable as early as 7 days and reached their maximal titres on day 21 (figure 2). Significant

* Health Animal Division of Solvay & Cie, Brussels.

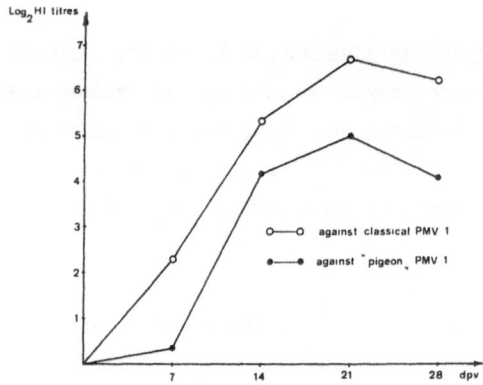

Fig. 2   Inactivated aqueous vaccine (LaSota strain): kinetic
of antibodies after vaccination.   (From Duchatel et al., 1985a).

differences were observed between the antibody titres according to whether
a classical PMV 1 strain or a "pigeon" PMV 1 strain was used in the HI
tests (figure 2; Duchatel et al., 1985a).   Titres were generally one or
two $\log_2$ less when reactions were performed against a "pigeon" PMV 1
strain.   Antibodies persisted at least 6 months after vaccination even when
titrated against a "pigeon" PMV 1 strain (figure 3; Duchatel et al., 1985b).
Ninety five to one hundred per cent of vaccinated pigeons resisted a severe
challenge performed 1 and 6 months after vaccination with either the Herts
33 strain or a "pigeon" PMV 1 strain (table 2; Duchatel et al., 1985a, b),
although the LaSota strain may be distinguished from the Herts 33 and the
"pigeon" strains with monoclonal antibodies prepared against the NDV
Ulster 2C strain (Russell and Alexander, 1983; Alexander et al., 1984).

TABLE 2   Vaccination trials with inactivated aqueous vaccine:
rates of morbidity-mortality after challenges.

Challenge strains	Months after vaccination	Morbidity-mortality	
		vaccinated pigeons	control pigeons
Herts 33/56	1	1/20	12/20
135/81 ("pigeon" strain)	1	0/20	18/20
135/81 ("pigeon" strain)	6	0/20	15/20

(From Duchatel et al., 1985a,b)

In comparison with control pigeons, vaccination also significantly reduced virus shedding in the laryngeal secretions and the faeces after challenge (figures 4, 5, 6, 7; Duchatel et al., 1985a, b).

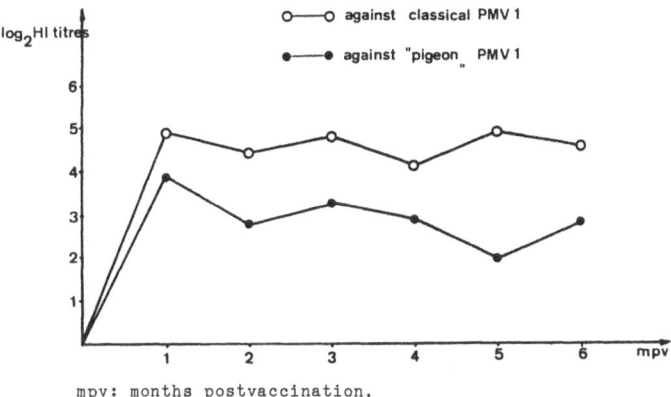

mpv: months postvaccination.

Fig. 3   Inactivated aqueous vaccine (LaSota strain): kinetic of antibodies after vaccination. (From Duchatel et al., 1985b).

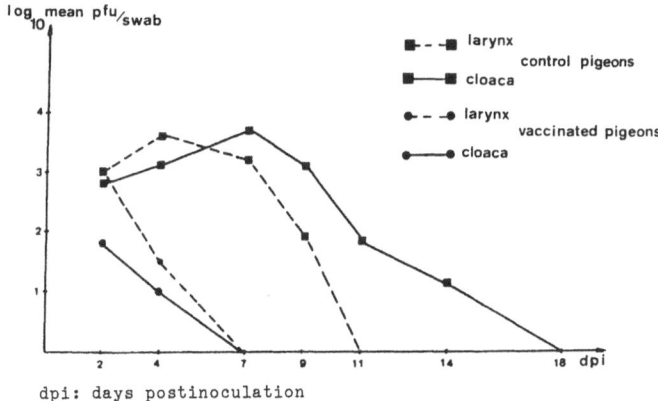

dpi: days postinoculation

Fig. 4   Inactivated aqueous vaccine (LaSota strain): means of numbers of viral particles excreted by control and vaccinated pigeons in the larynx and the cloaca after challenge with a "pigeon" PMV 1 strain 1 month post-vaccination. (From Duchatel et al., 1985a).

The efficacy of the inactivated aqueous suspension vaccine was compared to that of a commercial inactivated oil emulsion vaccine which contains inactivated Poletti strain (min. 50 PD 50) emulsified in an oil mineral adjuvant (0.5 ml pro dose 1). Sero-conversions were higher after injection of the aqueous vaccine than after injection of the oil vaccine

74

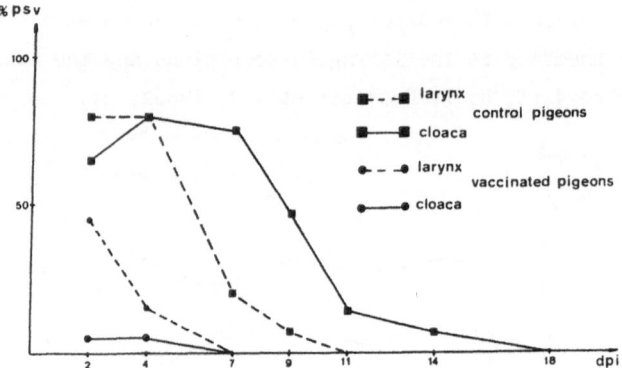

Fig. 5 Inactivated aqueous vaccine (LaSota strain): percentages of control and vaccinated pigeons which were shedding virus after challenge with a "pigeon" PMV 1 strain 1 month post-vaccination. (From Duchatel et al., 1985a).

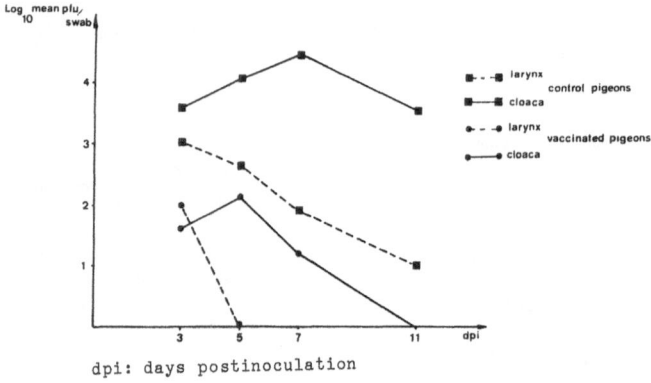

dpi: days postinoculation

Fig. 6 Inactivated aqueous vaccine (LaSota strain): means of numbers of viral particles excreted by control and vaccinated pigeons in the larynx and the cloaca after challenge with a "pigeon" PMV 1 strain 6 months post-vaccination. (From Duchatel et al., 1985b).

(figure 8). Although the oil vaccine contains the Poletti strain, differences were also observed between the HI titres if measured against a classical or a "pigeon" PMV 1 strain (figure 8) (Duchatel and Vindevogel, 1985c). After challenge 1 month post-vaccination, the morbidity-mortality rate reached 30% in the group of pigeons vaccinated with the oil vaccine and 100% in the control group. In contrast, no pigeon vaccinated with the aqueous vaccine developed symptoms of the disease (table 3).

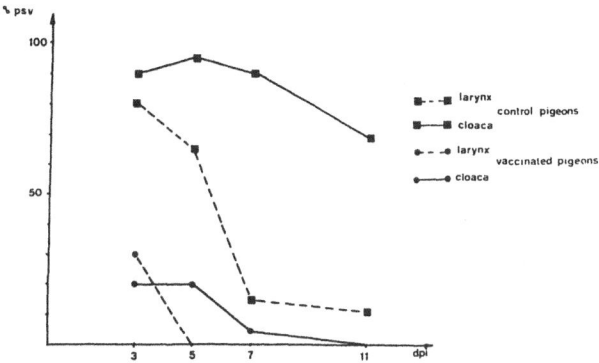

Fig. 7   Inactivated aqueous vaccine (LaSota strain): percentages
of control and vaccinated pigeons which were shedding virus after
challenge with a "pigeon" PMV 1 strain 6 months post-vaccination.
(From Duchatel et al., 1985b).

TABLE 3   Comparison between inactivated aqueous vaccine (LaSota
strain) and inactivated oil emulsion vaccine (Poletti
strain): rates of morbidity-mortality after challenge with
a "pigeon" strain 1 month post-vaccination.

Challenge strain	control group	vaccinated group (oil vaccine)	vaccinated group (aqueous vaccine)
135/81	20/20	6/20	0/20

(From Duchatel and Vindevogel, 1985c).

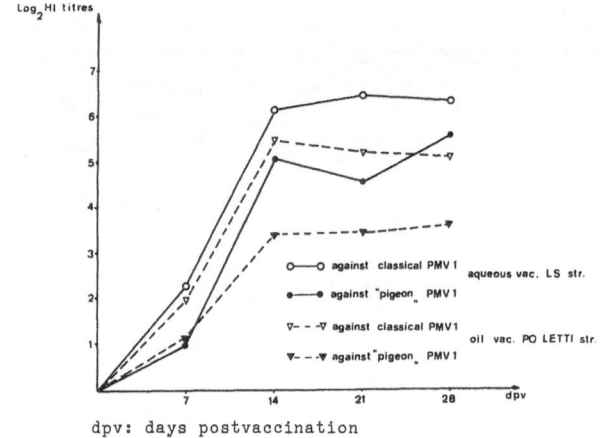

dpv: days postvaccination

Fig. 8   Comparison between inactivated aqueous vaccine (LaSota strain)
and inactivated oil emulsion vaccine (Poletti strain): kinetics of
antibodies after vaccinations. (From Duchatel and Vindevogel, 1985c).

REFERENCES

Alexander, D.J., Russell, P.H. and Collins, M.S. 1984. Paramyxovirus type
    1 infections of racing pigeons: 1 Characterisation of isolated viruses.
    Vet. Rec., 114, 444-446.
Chalmers, G.A. 1985. Personal communication.
Duchatel, J.P., Leroy, P., Coignoul, F., Pastoret, P.P. and Vindevogel, H.
    1985a. Essais de vaccination de pigeons contre la paramyxovirose par
    injection sous-cutanée de vaccins inactivés. Ann. Méd. Vét., 129,
    39-50.
Duchatel, J.P., Leroy, P. and Vindevogel, H. 1985b. Durée de la protection
    après vaccination de pigeons contre la paramyxovirose par injection
    sous-cutanée d'un vaccin inactivé aqueux (Colombovac PMV*). Preprint.
Duchatel, J.P. and Vindevogel, H. 1985c. Vaccination trials of pigeons
    against paramyxovirus type 1 infection with commercial or experimental
    inactivated aqueous or oil emulsion vaccines. Preprint.
Erickson, G.A., Brugh, M. and Beard, C.W. 1980. Viscerotropic velogenic
    Newcastle disease in pigeons: clinical disease and immunization.
    Avian Dis., 24, 257-267.
Guittet, M. and Bennejean, G. 1984. La paramyxovirose du pigeon.
    L'Aviculteur, 445, 59-62.
Heil, U. 1984. Untersuchungen zur charakterisierung und Klassifizierung
    des "Tauben-Paramyxovirus" sowie Überprüfung der Schutzwirkung
    verschiedener Newcastle-Disease- Impfstoffe bei Tauben (Columbia
    livia Gmel. 1789 var. dom.). Inaugural dissertation, Ludwig-
    Maximilians-Universität München.
Landré, F., Vindevogel, H., Pastoret, P.P., Schwers, A., Thiry, E. and
    Espinasse, J. 1982. Fréquence de l'infection du pigeon par le
    Pigeon herpesvirus 1 et le virus de la maladie de Newcastle dans le
    nord de la France. Rec. Méd. Vét., 158, 523-528.
Lumeji, J.T. and Stam, J.W.E. 1985. Paramyxovirus disease in racing pig-
    eons. Clinical aspects and immunization. A report from the

Netherlands. Vet. Quarterly, 7, 60-65.

Mousa, S., Ibrahim, A. and Shahata, M. 1982. Doves as carriers of Newcastle disease virus. Assiut Vet. Med. J., 10, 189-193.

Nunomura, M. 1984. Personal communication.

Richter, R., Kosters, J. and Kramer, K. 1983. Zur Paramyxovirus infektion bei Tauben. Prak. Tierarzt., 64, 915-918.

Russell, P.H. and Alexander, D.J. 1983. Antigenic variation of Newcastle disease virus strains detected by monoclonal antibodies. Arch. Virol., 75, 243-253.

Sabban, M.S., Zied, A.A., Basyouni, A., Nadiem, S., Barhouma, N. and Habashi, Y.Z. 1982. Susceptibility and possible role of doves in transmission of Newcastle disease in Egypt. Zentralbl. Vet., 29, 193-198.

Schusser, G., Lechner, C., Loupal, G., Wörgötter, J. and Vasicek, L. 1984. Paramyxovirus 1 infection in pigeons in Austria. Wiener Tierärztl. Monatssch., 71, 327-329.

Viaene, N., Spanoghe, L., Devriese, L., Bijnens, B. and Devos, A. 1983. Paramyxovirus bij duiven. Vl. Diergeneesk. T., 52, 278-286.

Vindevogel, H. 1981. Le coryza infectieux du pigeon. Thesis of "Agregation de l'Enseignement Supérieur", University of Liège, Faculty of Veterinary Medicine, Belgium.

Vindevogel, H. and Duchatel, J.P. 1985. Réactions post-vaccinales après injection de vaccin inactivé huileux contre la paramyxovirose chez le pigeon. Preprint.

Vindevogel, H., Duchatel, J.P., Coignoul, F., Leroy, P. and Pastoret, P.P. 1984. Essais de vaccination de pigeons contre la paramyxovirose au moyen de vaccins inactivés. Ann. Méd. Vét., 128, 643-649.

Vindevogel, H., Meulemans, G., Halen, P. and Schyns, P. 1972. Sensibilité du pigeon voyageur adulte au virus de la maladie de Newcastle. Ann. Rech. Vétér., 3, 519-532.

Vindevogel, H., Pastoret, P.P., Thiry, E. and Peeters, N. 1982a. Réapparition de formes graves de la maladie de Newcastle chez le pigeon. Ann. Méd. Vét., 126, 5-7.

Vindevogel, H., Pastoret, P.P., Thiry, E. and Calberg-Bacq, C.M. Ann. Méd. Vét., 127, 211-215.

Vindevogel, H., Thiry, E., Pastoret, P.P. and Meulemans, G. 1982b. Lentogenic strains of Newcastle disease virus in pigeons. Vet. Rec., 110, 497-499.

VACCINATION OF PIGEONS WITH LIVE AND INACTIVATED
VACCINES AGAINST PARAMYXOVIRUS-1 INFECTION

E.F. Kaleta*, B. Polten*, N. Schmeer**, J. Meister*
*Institut fur Geflugelkrankheiten
**Institut fur Hygiene und Infektionskrankheiten der Tiere
Justus-Leibig-Universitat
Frankfurter Str. 87
D-6300 Giessen
Federal Republic of Germany

ABSTRACT
    Comparative vaccination and challenge experiments with pigeons were
performed using mainly commercially available Newcastle disease vaccines
containing either live or inactivated antigen. The development of local
reactions (nodules) and increases in Chlamydia specific ELISA values following vaccination were used as parameters to gain information about the
innocuity of the vaccines. For the assessment of immunity the following
criteria were used (i) clinical symptoms, (ii) HI response in sera, (iii)
virus shedding in feces as assessed by cloacal swabs. Inactivated oil
emulsion vaccines induced local reactions at a rate between 0.5 and 2%.
Inactivated vaccines containing other adjuvants did not cause local reactions. All injected live virus vaccines containing aluminium hydroxide
gel were compatible following subcutaneous or intramuscular injection.
Live virus vaccines induced a more frequent increase in Chlamydia psittaci
specific ELISA values than inactivated vaccines. HI responses following
live virus vaccines were very low in comparison to inactivated vaccines.
Challenge experiments indicated differences in the rate of protection due
to vaccination with either live or inactivated vaccines.

INTRODUCTION

    Paramyxovirus-type 1 (PMV-1) infection is a widespread, very contag-

ious disease of pigeons. It occurs mainly in racing (carrier) pigeons and

also in other breeds such as show pigeons. It seems probable that other

species of the Order Columbiformes are also susceptible. Evidence of in-

fection has been noted following natural or experimental exposure in

chickens, turkeys, pheasants and other birds (Alexander et al., 1985).

    Although some control of the disease in domestic pigeons has been

achieved by measures to reduce the risk of lateral spread of the virus by

general sanitary measures, most success has arisen by the protection of

the susceptible pigeon population by vaccination. Initially, vaccines and

application procedures were used which were developed and approved to com-

bat Newcastle disease (ND) in the domestic chicken and turkey. It became

soon evident that mass vaccination procedures which are effective in

chickens failed to induce uniform and long-lasting protection in pigeon

lofts.

In this paper we describe the results of vaccination and challenge experiments with racing pigeons using injectable vaccines which contain either live or inactivated Newcastle disease viruses.

MATERIALS AND METHODS

Specified details on pigeons, vaccines and methods used are described elsewhere (Meister, 1985; Polten, 1985).

Pigeons

All pigeons originated from unvaccinated lofts of racing pigeons. They appeared clinically healthy and were free of detectable antibodies against the PMV-1 strain Montana in the hemagglutination inhibition test (HI test). All birds were examined daily for clinical symptoms to assess the innocuity of the vaccines and resistance to challenge.

Vaccines

Commercially available vaccines were mainly used. These included live virus vaccines containing B1 virus and aluminium hydroxide gel; the same adjuvant was also employed to prepare an experimental vaccine with LaSota type virus. Inactivated vaccines contained either mineral oil or carbomer as adjuvant. The live virus vaccines were injected intramuscularily using a volume of 0.5 ml, all inactivated vaccines were given subcutaneously in the neck.

HI test

Conventional techniques were used to detect antibodies in heat inactivated sera (microtitre system, 4 HA units of NDV strain Montana, 1 % chicken RBC).

ELISA

The ELISA technique for detection of antibodies against Chlamydia psittaci has been described elsewhere (Schmeer et al., 1984). Assays were performed with sera collected at the days of vaccination, challenge and necropsy, respectively.

Challenge

Intramuscular injection of a virulent strain of pigeon PMV-1 (de-

80

signated 1829/83) was used. Virus isolations were attempted from cloacal swabs up to three weeks following challenge using either embryonated hen's eggs or primary CEF cultures.

RESULTS

Innocuity of vaccines

The great majority of racing and show pigeons tolerated the injection of live and inactivated vaccines without any detectable adverse reaction. Improvements of the injection techniques and growing experience in handling large numbers of pigeons further reduced the number of undesired incidences. Although the frequency of fatalities associated with poor injection techniques has markedly decreased in recent years, a low level of accidents still occurs. These may be traced back to either the vaccine or to the pigeon itself.

It is a general impression that oil emulsion vaccines induce local swellings at the site of inoculation with an incidence between 0.5 to 2 %. These estimates are made by veterinary surgeons who vaccinate many thousands of pigeons in every season. The exact nature, eg. granuloma, abscess or others remains undetermined in most cases because spontaneous regression occurs within several weeks.

Some breeds of show pigeons have large dorsal diverticula of the crop which may be punctured with the needle. Injection at the lowest fourth of the neck may injure extensions of the air sacs.

Apoplectiform fatalities may also occur within one to a few hours post injection. In these cases aberrant venous connections between the left and right jugular veins are punctured. This results in extended bleeding and death due to anemia and/or shock.

Probable exacerbation of latent ornithosis by vaccination

In natural outbreaks of PMV-1 infection pigeons were occasionally seen which displayed uni- or bilateral conjunctivitis with serous-foamy lacrimal fluids. It is as yet undetermined whether this is a further PMV-1 associated manifestation or a chlamydia-induced symptom.

Many reports delineate the frequent reactivation of latent infection of pigeons with Chlamydia psittaci. We have been able to induce increases in Chlamydia-antibody titres following PMV-1 infection of PMV-1 susceptible pigeons ELISA latently infected with Chlamydia. A

similar increase in ELISA values could not be constantly induced by injecting oil emulsion vaccines containing inactivated NDV. It was desirable to
know whether injectable live virus vaccines behave similarily. Unfortunately this was not the case. Both B1 and also LaSota viruses induced in the
majority of latently infected (low titre) pigeons a drastic rise in Chlamydia ELISA values within 3 - 5 weeks post vaccination. The increase of
Chlamydia antibody titres was dependent on the dose of B1 or LaSota viruses (Table 1). Although symptoms of an apparent ornithosis could not be
produced in the experimental pigeons, we believe that any exacerbation
which may result in overt ornithosis must be considered as an undesireable
side effect of a live virus vaccine.

Response of pigeons to vaccination

The HI response of young pigeons one to four weeks following the first
injection of a B1 live virus adjuvanted vaccine is below the level of detection in almost all birds (Tables 2 and 3). A second injection of the
same type of vaccine induces a low level HI response of short duration
(Table 3). Under similar experimental conditions, all inactivated vaccines induce detectable and persisting antibodies in most pigeons (Table 3).

TABLE 1   Influence of the titre of B1 or LaSota live viruses in
injected vaccines on increment of Chlamydia psittaci
specific antibody values.

Vaccination $\log_{10}$ with EID_{50}/bird		Number of pigeons	Days post vaccination	Mean Chlamydia-specific antibody ELISA value (values of < 100 are con-sidered as non-specific)
B1	8.4	7	0	100
			42	390
B1	7.7	15	0	40
			31	250
B1	6.4	8	0	60
			42	50
B1	4.4-2.4	15	0	70
			42	60
LaSota	7.4	10	0	100
			31	390
none	--	25	0	30
			31-42	90

TABLE 2 Dose response of pigeons to intramuscular vaccination with B1 live virus adjuvant vaccine.

B1 virus $\log_{10}$ per pigeon	n	No. of pigeons with PMV-1 HI $(\log_2)$ p.vac. < 2	> 2	p.chal. < 2	> 2	No. of diseased pigeons post challenge	Cloacal swabs: virus pos.	total	%pos.
8.4	8	7	1	4	4	1	1	77	1.3
6.4	8	8	0	3	5	2	3	78	3.9
4.4	7	7	0	1	6	3	10	69	14.5
2.0	8	8	0	0	8	3	19	77	24.7
none	17	-	-	0	17	15	33	152	21.7

The rate of seroconversion is dependent on the amount of inactivated antigen given (Table 4).

The cloacal excretion of vaccinal B1 virus was monitored in a total of 53 pigeons which were intramuscularly vaccinated with different amounts of B1 virus. None of the 488 cloacal swabs from 53 pigeons contained detectable levels of B1 virus (Table 5) in primary and subcultures.

TABLE 3 Comparison of efficacy of live adjuvant and inactivated emulsion vaccines in pigeons.

Vaccines	n	No. of pigeons with PMV-1 HI $(\log_2)$ after 1.vac < 2	> 2	2.vac < 2	> 2	chal. < 2	> 2	Diseased pigeons p.chal. n	%	Cloacal swabs: virus pos.	total	%pos
1 x live adjuvant	26	24	2			7	19	7	26.5	13	248	5.2
1 x in-activated	45	8	37			0	45	4	8.9	13	493	2.6
live adjuvant + inactiv.	10	10	0	0	10	0	10	1	10.0	4	65	6.2
2 x live adjuvant	20	20	0	4	16	0	20	3	15.0	8	142	5.6
2 x in-activated	25	3	22	0	25	0	25	1	4.0	5	177	2.8
none	9	9	0	9	0	0	9	9	100.0	23	73	31.5

TABLE 4 Dose response of pigeons to subcutaneous vaccination
with inactivated emulsion vaccine.

Antigen content	n	No. of pigeons with PMV-1 HI ($\log_2$) p.vac.		p.chal.		No. of diseased pigeons post challenge	Cloacal swabs: virus		
		< 2	> 2	< 2	> 2		pos.	total	%pos.
undiluted	20	0	20	0	20	0	5	226	2.2
1 : 4	10	1	9	0	10	0	4	110	3.6
1 : 16	9	1	8	0	9	0	0	99	0
1 : 64	10	6	4	0	9	1	10	110	9.1
Placebo	9	9	0	0	9	9	31	99	31.3

The HI titre also gives an indication whether a pigeon will resist challenge or not. The likelihood of resistance to challenge increases with higher serum HI antibodies. This has been observed for live and inactivated vaccines (Table 6).

TABLE 5 Failure to detect vaccinal B1 virus in cloacal swabs of pigeons which were intramuscularly vaccinated with different amounts of B1 virus adsorbate vaccine.

Vaccination with $\log_{10}$ EID_{50}/bird		Number of pigeons	Sampling time days post vacc.	Number of B1 virus isolations pos./total tested
B1	7.3	11	2 - 12	0/110
B1	8.4	8	2 - 10	0/ 72
B1	6.4	8	2 - 10	0/ 72
B1	4.4	8	2 - 10	0/ 72
B1	2.4	8	2 - 10	0/ 72
B1	0.0	8	2 - 10	0/ 72
B1	7.7	10	2 - 11	0/ 90

Results of challenge experiments

Intramuscular challenge with approximately 10^8 EID_{50}/bird of the virulent 1829/83 pigeon PMV-1 results in an elevation of serum HI titres in almost all vaccinated pigeons. The probability of disease following challenge decreases with increasing HI titres on the day of challenge (Table 6).

84

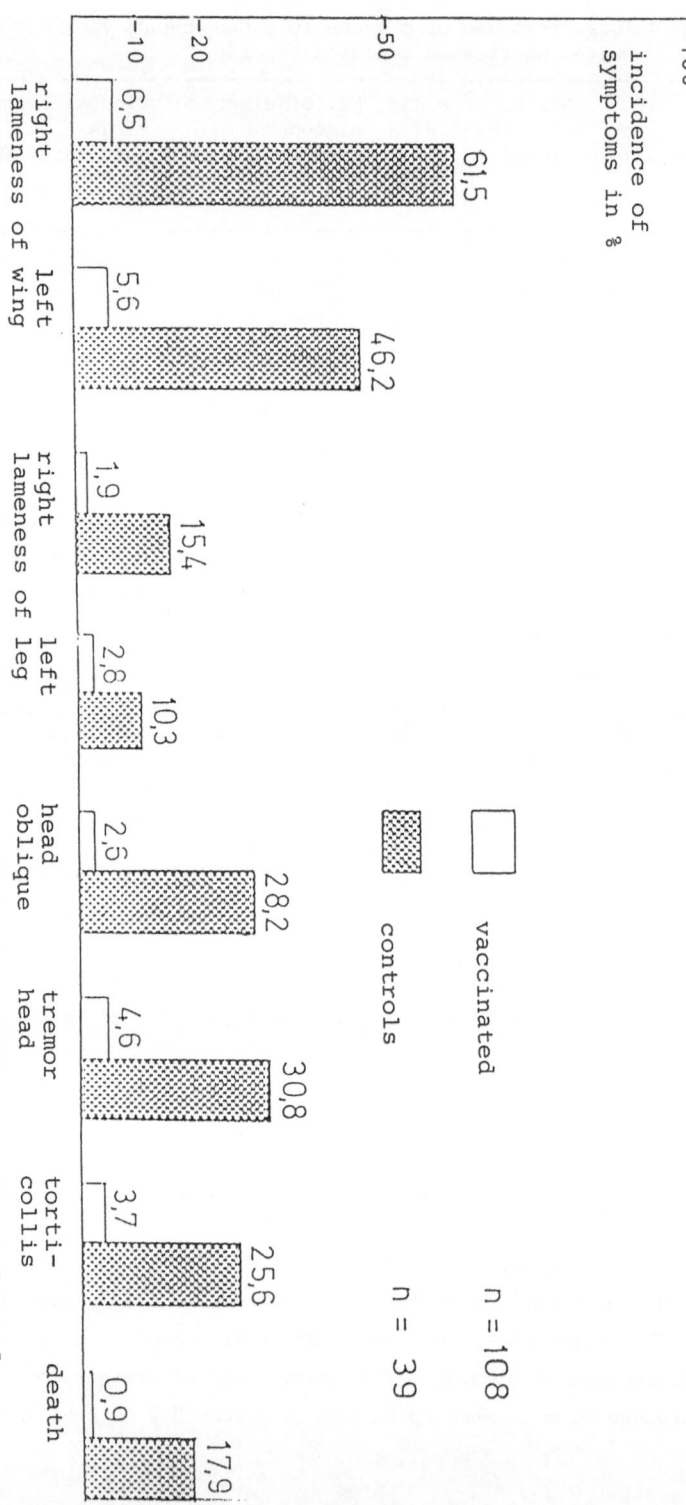

Fig. 1 Incidence of diverse clinical symptoms following challenge of vaccinated (inactivated vaccines only) and not vaccinated pigeons. A pigeon may exhibit several symptoms at the same time.

TABLE 6 Relationship between serum HI titres and resistance to
challenge of pigeons vaccinated either with live or
inactivated ND vaccines.

Vaccines	Outcome of challenge	Number of pigeons with HI titre ($\log_2$) at day of challenge							Total
		< 2	2	3	4	5	6	7	
live	diseased	21	2	2					25
viruses	healthy	46	10	9	10	2	1		78
inactivated	diseased	7	1	1	1				10
viruses	healthy	38	13	15	26	5	1	2	100

The immunizing capacity of the live B1 vaccine depends on the amount
of antigen given. The results in Table 2 indicate quite clearly that decreasing doses of vaccinal virus result in less protection against clinical
symptoms and virus excretion in feces. Similar effects can be noted with
an inactivated vaccine as shown in Table 4.

Although all vaccines used induced protection against challenge, none
of them was able to entirely prevent a clinical overt disease and excretion
of the challenge virus (Tables 2, 3 and 4). Comparison of the frequency of
clinical symptoms following challenge in vaccinated with unvaccinated controls indicates a reduction of incidence of specific symptoms (Fig. 1).
This demonstrates that the vaccinates are protected equally well against
lesions in the central as well as in the peripheral nervous system.

DISCUSSION

Both live and inactivated vaccines may protect against intramuscular
challenge with virulent pigeon PMV-1 virus. Two vaccinations spaced 4 - 6
weeks apart from each other do (only slightly) enhance the level of protection.

None of the live and inactivated vaccines used were able to prevent
disease or excretion of challenge virus. Increasing the amount of antigen did increase the level of protection.

High amounts of live viruses in vaccines result in an increase in
Chlamydia-specific ELISA values which are interpreted as an activation of
a latent infection by Chlamydia psittaci.

It seems to be desirable to replace conventional virulent or avirulent Newcastle disease viruses in inactivated vaccines by homologous

pigeon PMV-1 virus.

REFERENCES

Alexander, D.J., Russell, P.H., Parsons, G., Abu Elzein, E.M.E.,
     Ballouh, A., Cernik, K., Engstrom, B., Fevereino, M., Fleury, H.J.A.,
     Guittet, M., Kaleta, E.F., Kihm, U., Lomniczy, B., Meister, J.,
     Meulemans, G., Nerome, K., Petek, M., Polten, B., Prip, M., Richter,
     R., Sagi, E., Spanoghe, L. and Tumova, B. 1985. Antigenic and bio-
     logical characterization of avian paramyxovirus type 1 isolates from
     pigeons - an international collaborative study. Avian Pathol., 14,
     365-376.
Meister, J. 1985. Suz Paramyxovirus-1 Infektion der Tauben. Vet. Med.
     Diss. Giessen, in preparation.
Polten, B. 1985. Untersuchungen zur Schutzimpfung von Tauben gegen die
     Paramyxovirus-1-Infektion mit Vakzinen, die vermehrungsfahiges bzw.
     inaktiviertes Newcastle Disease-Virus enthalten. Vet. Med. Diss.
     Giessen, in preparation.
Schmeer, N., Meister, J., Kaleta, E.F., Polten, B. 1984. Ist Chlamydia
     psittaci ein komplizierender Faktor bei der Paramyxovirus-1-Infektion
     der Tauben? Dtsch. tierarztl. Wschr., 91, 398-399.

AVIAN PARAMYXOVIRUS TYPE 1 INFECTIONS IN PIGEONS - SPREAD
TO DOMESTIC POULTRY IN GREAT BRITAIN IN 1984

D.J. Alexander
Poultry Department
Central Veterinary Laboratory
New Haw, Weybridge, Surrey
KT15 3NB. United Kingdom

I.DISEASE IN PIGEONS

a)   Clinical signs

Although pigeons *(Columba livia)* and other members of the dove
family, *Columbidae,* have long been known to be susceptible to infection
with avian paramyxovirus type 1 (PMV-1) viruses, reports of natural infections have been rare and usually occurred when Newcastle disease has
been prevalent in domestic poultry (reviewed by Lancaster and Alexander,
1975).

In 1981 a disease of racing and show pigeons was first seen in
Europe and shown to be caused by a PMV-1 virus (Vindevogel *et al,* 1982).
Respiratory disease signs were notably absent in affected pigeons but
in all other respects the disease resembled the neurotropic form of Newcastle disease in chickens (Hanson, 1978). Clinical signs in pigeons
consisted of combinations of:- loss of condition, anorexia, excessive
drinking, diarrhoea (frequently green), torticollis, drooping of wings,
leg paralysis, alighting difficulties, tremors, inco-ordination and
abnormal flying. The number of signs seen and their severity varied
considerably but within these parameters the disease changed little
over the years 1981-1985. Mortality and even morbidity was often
difficult to assess due to culling by the owners and the very slow
spread within a loft. However in more severely affected lofts up to
80% of the birds showed signs of disease and mortality as high as 50%
was often reported. The disease appeared to be more severe in young
birds.

b)   Spread of disease

Reports of the disease suggest it first reached pigeons in Europe
in 1981 when it was seen in Italy (Perini *et al,* 1982). However there
is some evidence to suggest that the virus responsible was present in
Iraq in 1977 and that the clinical disease was seen in Egypt in early

1981 (Kaleta, personal communication).

Due to the mixing of birds from widespread geographical locations
at races and shows and trading of such birds, domesticated pigeons offer
an efficient means of propagation and spread of virus diseases. Between
1981 and 1984 virtually every European country reported the disease in
pigeons. In a collaborative study Alexander *et al* (1985a) examined
isolates from 15 different countries and confirmed their identity using
monoclonal antibodies (Table 1). In addition, reports from at least 9
other countries indicated the presence of disease. By 1984 the disease
of pigeons had reached panzootic proportions being reported in countries
representing Asia (Japan), Middle East (Iraq, Egypt, Israel), Africa
(Sudan) and North America (USA) in addition to the European countries.

The disease was first reported in Great Britain in July 1983, and
up to December 1983 disease was confirmed in 192 lofts (Alexander *et al*,
1984a). Vaccine was made available in September 1983, but there was a
marked reluctance to vaccinate susceptible pigeons. During 1984 further
spread of the disease was seen in racing and show pigeons and a total
of 866 outbreaks were confirmed (Alexander *et al*,1985c).

By the end of 1983 there was evidence in Great Britain (and other
European countries) that the disease had spread to feral pigeons. Although evidence of such infections was rare, a focus of disease at
Liverpool docks where large numbers of pigeons appeared to be severely
affected caused some concern. The pigeon population at Liverpool and
other docks in the Merseyside area was estimated as in excess of 30,000
birds and considerable numbers were seen to exhibit neurological signs
with associated high mortality. Virus was isolated from a carcase
submitted from this source in February 1984.

c)   Characterisation of isolates

Use of conventional polyclonal antiserum confirmed that the causi-
tive virus of the disease in pigeons was a PMV-1 (or Newcastle disease
virus, NDV) which showed some variation from more classical strains and
could be regarded as a variant. Alexander *et al* (1984b) used mouse
monoclonal antibodies to further characterize pigeon isolates and
demonstrate their distinctiveness. Russell and Alexander (1983) had
used monoclonal antibodies prepared against NDV-Ulster 2C to divide 40
NDV isolates into eight groups on the basis of their ability to cause
binding of the monoclonal antibodies to infected MDBK cells which they

and Alexander, 1983; Alexander *et al*, 1984b). This enabled a simple and rapid test to be employed to distinguish between pigeon isolates and most other PMV-1 viruses.

2. DISEASE IN DOMESTIC FOWL

a) Susceptibility of national flock

Vaccination against NDV infection had been made illegal in Great Britain from 1 September 1981. By 1984 the National poultry flock could be considered to be fully susceptible to NDV, although no outbreak of disease had been reported since vaccination had been stopped. In this respect Great Britain differed from the majority of mainland European countries where routine vaccination with live and dead vaccine continued to be practised.

b) Outbreaks in fowls

During February to July 1984 23 outbreaks of Newcastle disease were confirmed in domestic fowls in Great Britain (Alexander *et al*, 1985b)

The types of birds affected and the main clinical signs reported are summarized in Table 2. The main sign reported for egg-laying birds was characteristically egg production problems, beginning with white and soft-shelled eggs and gradually progressing to complete cessation of egg production in affected birds. In most cases diarrhoea was also present, with elevated mortality and nervous signs being reported occasionally.

In almost all outbreaks in laying birds spread of the disease was remarkably slow both within a house and from house to house. Several investigations on multihouse sites revealed that despite evidence of the virus being present for some weeks only a minority of the houses had infected birds.

In none of the three broilers flocks shown to be affected by the same virus as the egg-laying birds was diarrhoea reported. In these birds disease was first noticed as elevated and rising mortality associated with nervous signs consisting of difficulty in moving and eating, leg paralysis, weakness and lethargy. As with laying birds, spread was very slow and not all houses on a site were affected at the time of slaughter.

TABLE 1 Countries supplying PMV-1 viruses from pigeons antigenically
identical to British pigeon isolates[a]

Country[b]	Date of earliest isolate supplied
IRAQ	1977?
ITALY	24.12.81
SUDAN	7. 2.82
PORTUGAL	3. 8.82
FED. REP. GERMANY	20. 1.83
BELGIUM	28. 2.83
THE NETHERLANDS	24. 4.83
GREAT BRITAIN	21. 6.83
AUSTRIA	1983
CZECHOSLOVAKIA	27. 6.83
FRANCE	5. 7.83
HUNGARY	16. 7.83
DENMARK	5. 8.83
SWITZERLAND	29. 8.83
SWEDEN	12. 9.83
JAPAN	15.11.83
ISRAEL	1984

a: Data from Alexander *et al* (1985a)
b: Typical disease in pigeons has been reported from the following countries:- Egypt, 1981; Yugoslavia, 1982; Spain, 1983;
Malta, 1983; Cyprus, 1983; DRG, 1983; Poland, 1983; USA, 1984

assessed by an indirect immunoperoxidase test. It was shown that the
pigeon isolates represented a ninth distinct group of PMV-1 viruses.
The ability to distinguish unequivocally between the viruses responsible for the disease in pigeons and other PMV-1 viruses greatly aided
the diagnosis and epizootiological studies of the disease. Over 50
British pigeon isolates and over 50 isolates from pigeons from other
countries have been tested and all showed identical monoclonal antibody binding patterns (Alexander *et al*, 1985a). In addition, except for
four duck isolates, the pigeon isolates were the only viruses tested
which were not inhibited by the monoclonal antibodies directed against
the HN-1 epitope in haemagglutination inhibition (HI) tests (Russell

TABLE 2 Clinical signs reported in 23 outbreaks of Newcastle Disease in fowls in Great Britain in 1984[a]

Type of birds involved	Number of flock affected	Egg production problems	Nervous signs	Diarrhoea	Elevated mortality	Respiratory signs
Commercial layers	11	10	1	3	2	0
broiler breeders	6	6	3	2	1	0
broilers a)	3	–	3	0	3	0
b)	1[b]	–	0	1	1	1
backyard flocks of assorted poultry	2	0	0	0	0	0

a: Data from Alexander *et al* (1985b)

b: This broiler flock was not infected with pigeon PMV-1 virus

92

The disease signs in chickens in these outbreaks were similar to
those produced in experimental infections of chickens with PMV-1 viruses
isolated from pigeons. While the lack of respiratory signs and slowness
of spread were consistent with the suspected faecal/oral route of
infection.

The second outbreak of NDV to be confirmed was considered to be
unassociated with the other 22 (see below). In this outbreak, in broilers, the birds showed respiratory distress, diarrhoea and high mortality.
Morbidity was high, suggesting rapid spread. In addition to the isolation of NDV of relatively low virulence, the birds were experiencing an
Escherichia coli problem.

c) Characterization of isolated viruses

Viruses, shown to be PMV-1 by conventional polyclonal chicken
antiserum, were isolated from all outbreaks, with the exception of two
backyard flocks in contact with the first outbreak and shown to be
serologically positive. With the exception of virus from outbreak 2,
all virus isolates were shown to have identical monoclonal antibody
binding patterns to the PMV-1 viruses isolated from pigeons (Table 3).
In addition, again with the exception of virus from outbreak 2, these
viruses were not inhibited in HI tests with monoclonal antibodies
directed against the HN-1 epitope.

During investigations into the disease outbreaks it was necessary
to exclude possible spread from NDV infections of psittacines which
occurred on quarantine premises at the end of 1983 and beginning of
1984. Viruses isolated from these sources also showed quite different
monoclonal binding patterns and HI titres with the HN-1 monoclonal
antibodies (Table 3).

d) Sources of infection

The use of monoclonal antibodies established the virus from the
first outbreak in chickens as identical to the PMV-1 virus affecting
pigeons and that the most likely source of infection was from diseased
pigeons. However in the first and all subsequent outbreaks contact
with racing pigeons seemed very unlikely and contact with feral pigeons could only be considered as a possibility in one or two of the
outbreaks. Epizootiological tracing for the first outbreak revealed
that constituents of the rations fed to the birds came from stores at

TABLE 3   Characterization of PMV-1 viruses from pigeons and poultry

| Isolates | HI titres with: | | monoclonal antibody binding pattern[a] |
	chicken serum	monoclonal antibody to HN-1[a]	
1983/4 British pigeon isolates	64–256	<10	p
pigeon isolates from other countries	64–512	<10	p
British chicken isolates from outbreaks 1, 5– 23	128–512	<10	p
chicken outbreak 2	1024	640	e
feral pigeons at Liverpool docks (2)	256–512	<10	p
carcases in food at Liverpool docks	256	<10	p
food at Liverpool docks (2)	256	<10	p
psittacine isolates (2)	512–1024	320–640	c
NDV-B1	1024	640	e
NDV-F	1024	640	f
Ulster 2C	512	640	g

a: See:- Russell and Alexander (1983) Alexander *et al* (1985a)

Liverpool docks that were infested with diseased pigeons. Examination of the stores of ingredients for chicken food at Liverpool and associated docks revealed the presence of pigeon carcases, feathers and avian faeces in the food. PMV-1 viruses were isolated from pigeon carcases taken from the food and from samples of the food itself.

The association of outbreaks in chickens with food from Liverpool docks was strong, especially as subsequent outbreaks showed links with this source. However the implications of this as a source of virus are that virus would survive any storage period, the milling process and that chickens would become infected if virus was presented in this way. The first and third points have been shown experimentally, since it has been demonstrated that NDV will survive for periods of six months or more in avian faeces under normal temperatures (Lancaster, 1956) and Alexander *et al* (1984c) have shown that chickens become infected when fed food artificially contaminated with infectious pigeon faeces. In Britain it is the practice to feed layer and broiler breeder hens on rations which are merely mixed at the mills and untreated in any other way. This point seemed to be extremely important in the epizootiology of the outbreaks, as other birds are usually fed pelleted food. Pelleting involves a brief heating process in which temperatures of about 80°C are held for up to 30 seconds. The inference is that this is sufficient to kill the PMV-1 virus as no primary outbreaks occurred in birds receiving pelleted food.

Eight of the 23 outbreaks were in birds fed rations known to contain ingredients from pigeon-infested stores at Liverpool or associated docks. A further six outbreaks were in birds which received rations probably contaminated with food from these stores. Five outbreaks were probably due to spread by direct contact with infected premises. Two of these were broiler flocks that had received chicks hatched from eggs from affected hens, but Alexander *et al* (1985b) considered mechanical contamination, rather than vertical transmission, to be responsible for the disease in the progeny.

The source of virus for four outbreaks, including the unrelated outbreak, remained untraceable.

e)   Control

Legislation was invoked to restrict movement of contaminated food from premises at Liverpool and associated docks. A monitoring and inspection scheme aimed at prevention of wild bird infestation was also set up to prevent recurrence of the situation.

In keeping with the 'stamping out' policy that existed at the time, all birds on the affected sites were slaughtered and disposed of. This involved over 800,000 birds and a claim of over £2,000,000 was made against the industry-financed insurance scheme which applied at that time.

The last outbreak was confirmed in mid-July 1984 and no further
outbreaks have occurred in the eleven months up to the time of writing,
despite an increase in the outbreaks of disease in racing pigeons during
1984 (Alexander *et al,* 1985c) and the continued occasional evidence of
disease in wild birds. Notwithstanding the apparent success of the
control measures, Industry decided to discontinue financing the 'stamping out' policy insurance scheme and the national control policy for
NDV reverted to one of vaccination in September, 1984.

REFERENCES

Alexander, D.J., Wilson, G.W.C., Thain, J. and Lister, S.A. 1984a.
    Avian paramyxovirus type 1 infection of racing pigeons: 3
    epizootiological considerations. Vet. Rec., 115, 213-216.
Alexander, D.J., Russell, P.H. and Collins, M.S. 1984b. Paramyxovirus
    type 1 infections of racing pigeons: 1 characterization of isolated
    viruses. Vet. Rec., 114, 444-446.
Alexander, D.J., Parsons, G. and Marshall, R. 1984c. Infection of fowls
    with Newcastle disease virus by food contaminated with pigeon
    faeces. Vet. Rec., 115, 601-602
Alexander, D.J. and 25 others 1985a. Antigenic and biological charac-
    terization of avian paramyxovirus type 1 isolates from pigeons -
    an international collaborative study. Avian. Path., in press.
Alexander, D.J., Wilson, G.W.C., Russell, P.H., Lister, S.A. and
    Parsons, G. 1985b. Newcastle disease outbreaks in fowls in Great
    Britain during 1984. Vet. Rec., in press.
Alexander, D.J., Lister, S.A. and Wilson, G.W.C. 1985c. Avian paramyxo-
    virus type 1 infections of racing pigeons: 5 continued spread in
    1984, in preparation.
Hanson, R.P. 1978. Newcastle disease. In Diseases of Poultry Hofstad,
    M.S. ed. 7th ed. Iowa State Univ. Press: Ames p 513.
Lancaster, J.E. 1966. Newcastle disease a review- 1926-1964. Monograph
    No. 3 Canada Dept. Agriculture: Ottawa.
Lancaster, J.E. & Alexander, D.J. 1975. Newcastle disease - virus and
    spread. Monograph No. 11. Canada Dept. Agriculture : Ottawa.
Perini, S., Marastoni, G. and Pascucci, S. 1982. Sull'attuale epizooia
    di malattia di Newcastle nei piccioni. Selezione Vet., 23 129-130.
Russell, P.H. and Alexander, D.J. 1983. Antigenic variation of
    Newcastle disease virus strains detected by monoclonal antibodies.
    Archiv. Virol., 75, 243-253.
Vindevogel, H., Pastoret, P.P., Thiry, E. and Peeters, N. 1982. Re-
    apparition de formes graves de la maladie de Newcastle chez le
    pigeon. Ann. Med. Vet., 126, 5-7.

RECENT ADVANCES IN PARAMYXOVIRUS INFECTION OF TURKEYS IN FRANCE

F.X. Le Gros

Ministere de l'Agriculture - Direction de la Qualité
Services Vétérinaires
Laboratoire National de Pathologie Aviaire
22440, Ploufragan, France

ABSTRACT

Paramyxovirus (PMV) types 1, 2 or 3, are encountered in turkey flocks in France. Lentogenic PMV1 and PMV2 are associated with respiratory problems (Infectious Rhinotracheitis) but they do not seem to be the main etiological agents of this condition. PMV3 alone was detected in laying flocks associated with egg drops. A recently undertaken vaccination programme against PMV3 gives incomplete protection.

INTRODUCTION

Isolations of virus or serological studies undertaken during recent years have shown the presence of PMV1, 2 and 3 in turkey flocks in France. Two kinds of clinical signs are associated with these infections, namely respiratory or laying problems (Andral and Louzis, 1982; Andral and Toquin, 1984) as observed in other countries (Alexander, 1980; Lang et al., 1975; MacPherson et al., 1983).

PARAMYXOVIRUS AND RESPIRATORY TROUBLES

Newcastle disease (ND) has not been detected in France since 1975 in turkeys or other poultry. However, it is necessary to emphasise the comparative resistance of turkeys to NDV. For instance, the velogenic strain "Ploufragan" (ICPI 1.75, MDT : 50 h) which kills up to 100% of inoculated chickens within three days, does not produce any mortality in turkeys, but causes only slight prostration and anorexia around the 10th day post infection. Only a few birds show transient nervous signs, occasionally hemiplegia may result.

Therefore one must be very careful with turkey PMV1 isolates: a velogenic strain may not produce serious clinical signs. It is necessary to assess the pathogenicity of each isolated PMV1 by the standard tests using chickens and embryonated eggs. This has been done with PMV1 isolated in the field from 1981 to 1984 in outbreaks of infectious rhinotracheitis in turkeys, a disease which appeared in Brittany in June 1981. The six PMV1 isolates were classified as lentogenric viruses as shown in Table 1

(from Andral, 1984). Both virus and Chlamydia were invariably isolated together from this condition (Andral and Louzis, 1982; Andral et al., 1985).

TABLE 1   Comparative pathogenic features of various PMV1 isolates.

Strain	Hitchner B1	La Sota	PMV1 isolates	GB Texas
MDT	128	104	107 to 127	60
ICPI	0.1	0.2	≤ 0.1	1.8

The three PMV2 isolates, which were identified by cross HI tests
(Table 2) (from Andral, 1984) were like the six isolates of PMV1 apatho-
genic for turkeys. However, clouding of the air sacs is produced by experimental infection of two week old SPF turkeys with an inoculum containing PMV2 and Chlamydia psittaci (Andral, unpublished).

TABLE 2   Identification of three PMV2 isolates (HI test)

	Reference strain serum		
	PMV1	PMV2	PMV3
Homologous strain	> 640	> 640	> 640
Strain 83 373	10	640	10
" 83 387	20	1280	10
" 83 435	20	640	10

Seroconversion in the field with these viruses takes up to five weeks
to appear, and titres stay at low levels. Sometimes, seroconversion does
not occur in the whole flock, but in only a proportion. However, experimental infection of 24 SPF two week old turkeys with one of these PMV2
isolates gave a slight but clear response on the third week (Andral, unpublished), with a geometric mean titre of 1:25 $(2^{4.7}$; s : 2.17).

Figure 1 compares the experimental PMV2 HI antibody response to the
field one, obtained in the same 24 birds during the twelve weeks after
rhinotracheitis (from Metz-Toux, 1984). This illustrates the poor invasive-
ness of these PMV strains in natural infections and their unprobable
etiological rule in rhinotracheitis.

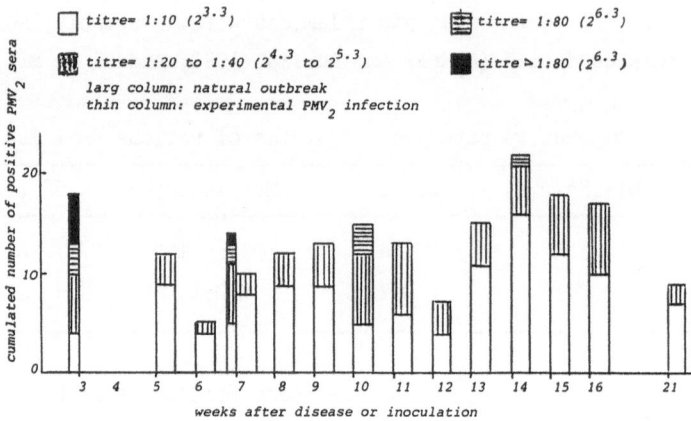

Fig. 1   Comparison of two anti-PMV2 serological responses (HI test).

PARAMYXOVIRUS AND EGG DROPS

In November 1982, the first positive serological responses were observed against PMV3 on a flock reared in Normandie. Then, in 1983, this occurred throughout France (Andral and Toquin, 1984). In these flocks, no respiratory symptoms were observed. Only laying problems consisting of egg drops associated with poor egg shell quality occurred. Since December 1983, four strains of PMV have been isolated from such flocks. Three of these were identified as PMV3. The remaining isolate was a PMV2 which was associated with a PMV3. In the latter case a serological response (HI test) was observed against PMV3, but not PMV2 (Andral, 1984).

With these egg drops, the antibody response against PMV3 was transient and occurred between the 3rd and 6th week after the disease. In flocks unvaccinated against ND, HI titres were low, about 1:30 (2^5), and not associated with an anti-PMV1 response. In flocks vaccinated against ND, the first response was against PMV1 and then anti-PMV3, with titres reaching to 1:80 ($2^{6.3}$), as observed by others (Alexander et al., 1983).

Figures 2, 3 and 4 (from Andral and Toquin, 1984) show the laying curves of three different flocks and their serological responses against PMV3. The last flock was vaccinated against ND. In the case of the last flock, the development of antibody titres suggests an endemic persistence of the virus on the farm, and the possibility of reinfection of this flock, or the next one, as observed in the field by other authors (Lang, reported by Andral and Toquin, 1984).

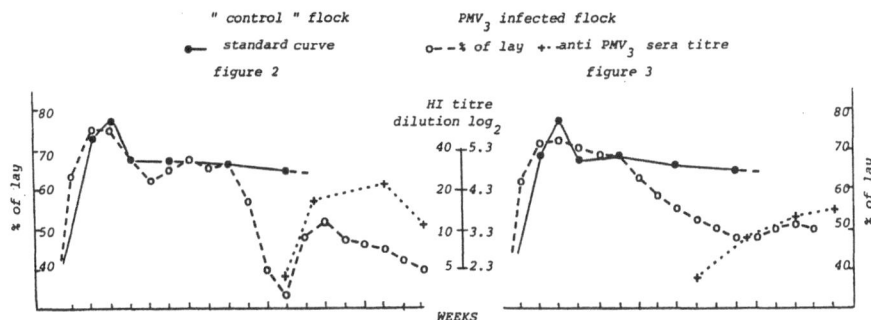

Figs 2 and 3. Laying curve and PMV3 antibody response (HI test): flocks unvaccinated against ND.

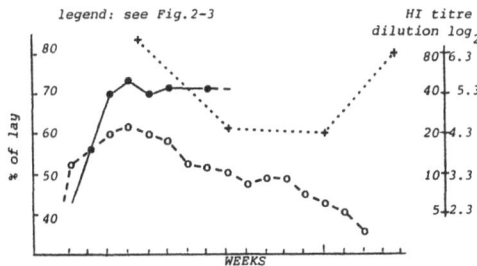

Fig 4. Laying curve and PMV3 antibody response (HI test): flock vaccinated against ND.

PMV3 vaccination was undertaken in the field during 1984. The vaccination schedule was as follows:
- 8th week: Pasteurellosis
- 12th week: Pasteurellosis + NDV (inactivated, oil adjuvant)
- 22th week: NDV + EDS76
          erysipelas
          PMV3 (inactivated, oil adjuvant)
- 26th week: erysipelas
          Fowl Pox
          PMV3 (inactivated, oil adjuvant)

The serological response usually obtained is shown in figure 5. Features to note are the short duration of the HI titres and the absence of booster effect after the second injection. At the beginning of lay, titres are 1:30 (2^5). Titres are based on the results from 30 turkeys hens. The typical response could be explained by insufficient time between the first and second injection (4 weeks) or an antagonism between erysipelas or fowl pox vaccine in the second injection of PMV3.

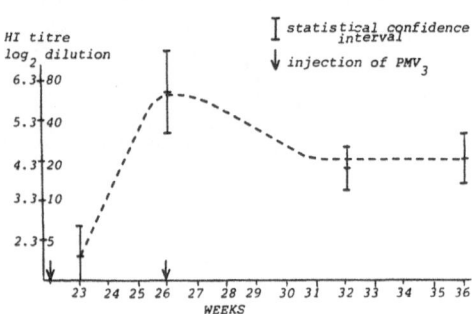

Fig 5.   Antibody response against PMV3 after vaccination.

These low titres suggest an incomplete protection resulting in slight laying troubles: egg drops of a few per cent, low point of lay, poorer egg shell quality. In figures 6, 7 and 8 three examples are given. In those flocks, the booster effect resulting from the natural infection is swift, after a short period when antibodies are consumed. The HI titres increase by about two dilutions (2 $\log_2$) within 2-3 weeks. Then they decrease quite quickly to their initial level, so that a further reinfection is possible.

The anti-PMV1 response can stay unchanged, or develop in a parallel manner to that against PMV3, as in Figure 8. In this outbreak, a PMV1 could have been suspected as the cause, but taking into account the high HI titres against PMV1, we could not explain such a negative effect on egg production.

In the first example a neighbouring flock, a few dozen meters distant and reared by the same farmers showed no change in its PMV3 antibody titres, showing the poor spreading aptitude of this virus.

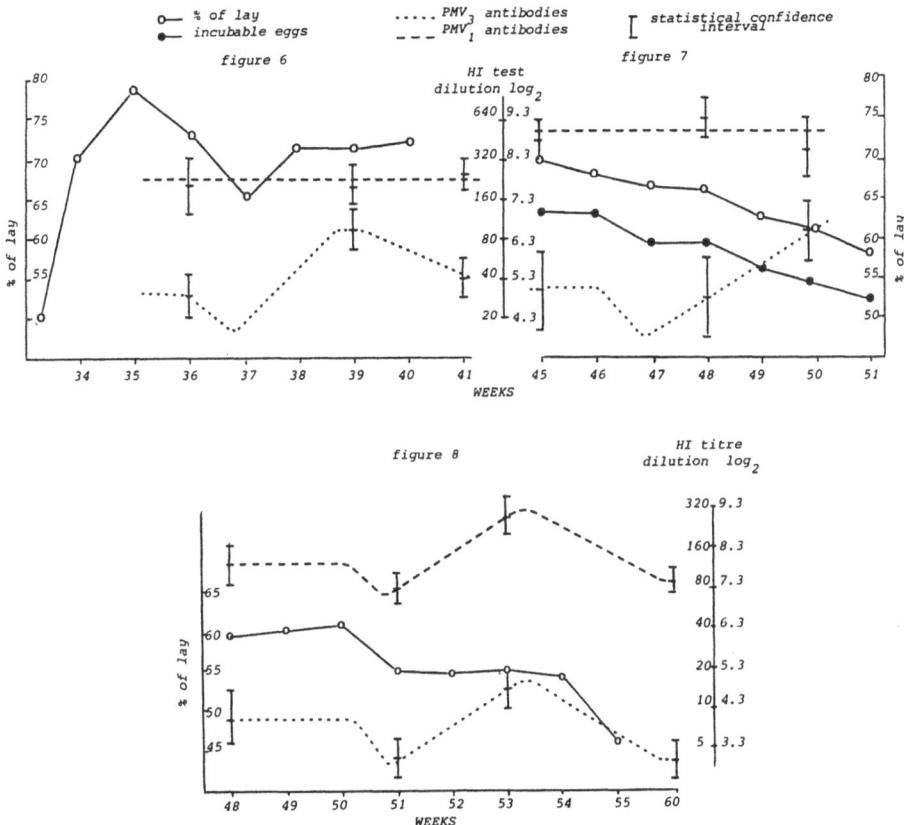

Figs 6, 7 and 8. Laying troubles in flocks vaccinated against PMV3 compared with their PMV3 antibody kinetics.

CONCLUSION

Although pathogenic strains of NDV are absent in France, paramyxovirus infections frequently occur in turkey flocks, as in other areas of the world with intensive production. Nevertheless, no primary etiological role can be attributed to PMV types 1 and 2 which can act as secondary agents in respiratory diseases. The negative effect of PMV3 infections on egg production is obvious. Hopefully, this will soon be controlled by vaccination.

REFERENCES

Alexander, D.J. 1980. Avian Paramyxovirus. Veterinary Bulletin, 50, 737-752.

Alexander, D.J., Pattison, M., MacPherson, I. 1983. Avian Paramyxoviruses of PMV3 serotype in British turkeys. Avian Pathology, 12, (4), 469-482.

Andral, B., Louzis, C. 1982. La rhinotrachéite de la dinde en Bretagne, Bull. Lab. Vet. 7, 33-43.

Andral, B. 1984. Les myxoviruses de la dinde en France. L'Aviculteur, 445, 67-73.

Andral, B., Toquin, D. 1984. Isolation of Avian PMV2 and 3 from turkeys in Brittany. Veterinary Record, 114, 570-571.

Andral, B., Toquin, D. 1984. Infection à Myxovirus: chutes de ponte chez les dindes reproductrices. 1. Infection par les PMV aviaires de type III. Recueil de Médecine Vétérinaire, 160, (1) 43-48.

Andral, B., Louzis, C., Newman, J.A., Toquin, D., Bennejean, J. 1985. Respiratory disease (rhinotracheitis) in turkeys in Brittany, France, 1981-1982. II Laboratory findings. Avian Diseases, 29, (1), 35-42.

Lang, G., Gagnon, A., Howell, J. 1975. Occurrence of PMV Yucaipa in Canadian poultry. Canadian Veterinary Journal, 16, 233-237.

MacPherson, I., Watt, R.G., Alexander, D.J. 1983. First isolation of an avian PMV other than Newcastle Disease virus from commercial poultry Great Britain. Veterinary Record, 112, 479-480.

ACKNOWLEDGEMENTS

We are very grateful to D. Toquin (Laboratoire National de Pathologie Aviaire) for his excellent technical work.

THE DIAGNOSIS AND CONTROL OF INFECTIOUS BRONCHITIS
VARIANT INFECTIONS

F.G. Davelaar, B. Kouwenhoven and A.G. Burger

Poultry Health Institute
P.O. Box 43, 3940 AA DOORN
The Netherlands

ABSTRACT

In this paper the diagnosis of IB infections is discussed. This is
based on clinical signs and laboratory examinations. The laboratory tests
can be divided into 2 groups.
A. Serological tests
   - agar gel precipitation test,
   - virus neutralization test,
   - haemagglutination inhibition test.
B. Demonstration of viral antigen
   - immunofluorescence test,
   - virus isolation and identification.
Using these techniques the following programme is used to control IB:
1. Inventory of the incidence of IB infections.
2. Virus isolation and serotyping; monitoring of incidence.
3. Development of vaccines.
4. Evaluation of the vaccination programme.
Implementation of this programme has resulted in a sharp decrease of IB
infections in The Netherlands.

INTRODUCTION

Despite vaccination against Infectious Bronchitis virus (IBV), infection of poultry with this virus still causes disease problems in many countries. Entitled with the common name Infectious Bronchitis (IB), disease
symptoms vary greatly from respiratory distress in young birds to a peak
of egg production below predicted levels, depressed production, shell abnormalities and intercurrent diarrhoea in laying and parent stock or a
combination of these symptoms.

In the Netherlands IB is controlled mainly by vaccination with the
live attenuated vaccine viruses H120 and H52. Since 1976 vaccination with
the more attenuated H120 vaccine virus has been carried out mainly by
application as a coarse droplet spray to newly hatched chicks. The less
embryo-adapted H52 vaccine virus is subsequently applied, perferably by eye
drop, at an age of about 15 to 18 weeks. The immunological basis for the
day-old spray application has been published before (Davelaar et al.,
1982).

The H120 and H52 vaccines based on the H-strain originally isolated by Bijlenga et al. (1956) are up to the present the best option for a vaccine against IB since these vaccines have a wide antigenic spectrum. Winterfield (1975) showed that many, although not all, of the IBV strains isolated in the USA from birds suffering from respiratory and/or production problems (these strains to be distinguished from those causing kidney problems, such as the Holte, Gray and Australian T strains), were immunologically "covered" well by the H-vaccine.

It was therefore surprising that the improved results achieved by the newly introduced improved vaccinations were not consistent (text fig. 3).

From 1979 an increasing number of properly vaccinated flocks suffered from respiratory (mainly broilers) and from egg production problems as described. In many of these cases IB was diagnosed by a combination of serology (rise in HI titers and numbers of birds reacting in the AGP test), demonstration of IBV antigen with the direct immunofluorescence test (IFT) in frozen tracheal sections and virus isolation.

In this paper the significance of clinical observation and of laboratory tests to diagnose IB will be discussed. Thereafter the design and the results of our study on the situation in the Netherlands are presented.

DIAGNOSIS

Clinical signs

In practice IB in young chicks is diagnosed on respiratory signs. In adult birds IB problems are manifested by either dramatically decreased egg production with typical egg shell problems and occasionally respiratory problems or by failure to reach peak production or by depressed production, or by a combination of the signs. In many cases however, due to a lack of obvious signs, there is a need for a definitive diagnosis by laboratory tests. These tests are based on the demonstration of antibody (serology) or on the presence of the viral antigen (immunofluorescence and isolation).

Serological tests

 - The agargel precipitation (AGP) test (Woernle, 1959).
With this type of test precipitating antibodies can be demonstrated in blood or serum. A couple of weeks after infection the concentration of precipitating antibodies reaches its peak and declines thereafter. In other words, shortly after infection a high percentage of AGP positive sera will be found, whereas about one month later a clear decline in the

number of positive reactors appears. In the test the group antigen of
the avian coronaviruses is detected and the test is therefore not serotype specific.

  - Virus neutralization test.
The virus neutralization (VN) test in embryonated SPF eggs (alpha method)
used to classify IBV isolates and to detect antibody in poultry flocks has
been described by Lukert (1975). The test is serotype specific.

  - Haemagglutination inhibition test (HI-test) (Alexander and Chettle,
1977).
IBV is able, after treatment with the enzyme phospholipase - C, to bind
with erythrocytes (= haemagglutination). By incubating the virus with
antiserum, the haemagglutination can be blocked. By testing antisera in
twofold dilutions against the haemagglutination inhibition ability, the
antibody-titer can be determined.

  We have demonstrated that the HI test is serotype-specific.
Text figure 1 shows that the homologous HI titer after a single eye
drop inoculation of chicks with the D274 isolate is high after 2

TEXT FIGURE 1

HI
(Log base 2)

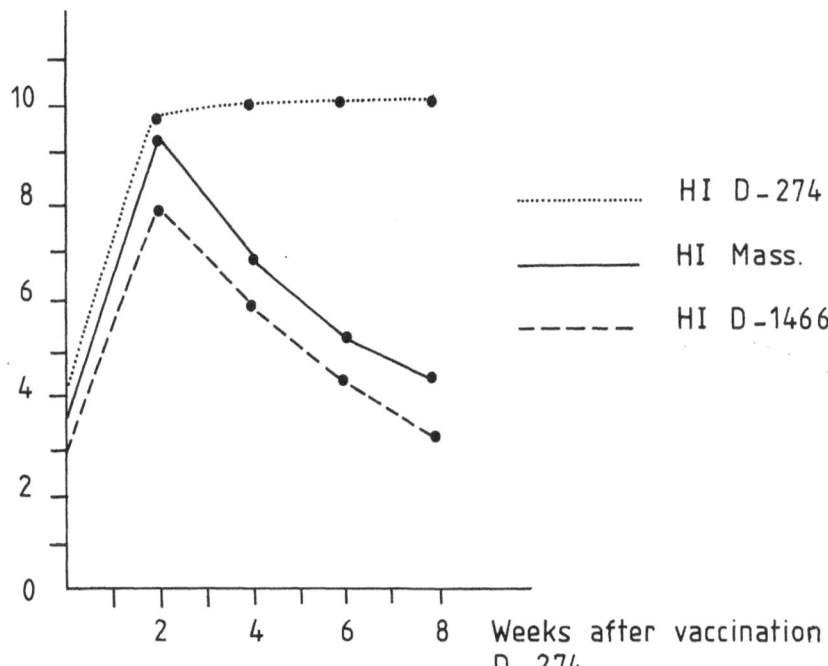

weeks and persists at the same level until the end of the experiment. HI
titers measured with antigens of the Massachusetts and the D1466 serotypes
peak 2 weeks after inoculation and decline thereafter. So group-specific
reactions occur only for a short time after inoculation. Table 1 represents the results of cross HI tests carried out with sera obtained 5 weeks
after inoculation. The results show the relative type-specificity of the
HI tests.

TABLE 1   HI experiment demonstrating the type difference between
the new isolates (Titer expressed as $\log_2$).

Serum \ Virus (Type)	M41 (Mass)	D274 (207)	D1466 (212)
H52 (Mass)	9	6	5
207	6	10	5
212	5	5	8
246G (Mass)	10	5	n.d.

Demonstration of viral antigen

- Immunofluorescence test (IFT).

With this technique IBV can be visualized in cryostat sections by reacting
the virus antigens with fluorescent antibody (conjugate). Usually IBV can
be demonstrated in the trachea up to 10 to 14 days after infection. The
test is not serotype specific but reacts with the group antigen of the avian coronaviruses.

- Virus isolation and identification.

In our study IBV was primarily isolated from tracheal samples, even in
cases of egg production problems without evident respiratory symptoms. In
a later stage of the study we found that including the upper part of the
caeca containing the caecal tonsils increased the isolation scores greatly.

However, a comparison between isolation from trachea and caeca has not
been carried out. Freshly collected tracheal samples (appr. 3 cm long)
from 3 to 5 birds from an affected flock were cut in longitudinal slices
and ground together with the upper caeca from the same birds in a mortar
and pestle with sterile sand after addition of cold sterile saline to make

up an organ suspension of about 10 volume per cent. Tracheas are not completely macerated by this treatment but it yields a suspension of sufficient
mucous membrane in saline. After grinding, the suspension was centrifuged
for 30 mins at 3000 g and 4°C. The supernatant was incubated for 30 mins
at 4°C with 5 mg Streptomycin and 5000 IU Penicillin per ml and then 0.2 -
1 ml was inoculated into the allantoic cavity of each of 5, 8-10 days embryonated eggs from a specific pathogen free (SPF) flock. Eggs were candled daily. Embryo mortality within 24 hours after inoculation was regarded as non-specific.

When embryo mortality or embryonic changes (dwarfing, clubbed down)
had not occurred by day 6 after inoculation, eggs were cooled overnight at
4°C. One ml volumes allantoic fluid were collected from each embryo the next
day, pooled, incubated with antibiotics and inoculated into the allantoic
cavity of five other embryos as before. This procedure was repeated three
more times (total 5 embryo passages of the suspected suspension) before a
sample was regarded as negative. It should be remarked that in some ex-
ceptional cases up to 12 passages had to be made before a virus was isolated.

When embryo changes or embryo mortality was observed, the chorioallantoic membranes (CAM) of the infected embryos were collected, blotted
with tissue and small pieces were minced and examined in an AGP test with
monospecific precipitating fowl antisera against IBV, REO virus, Adenovirus,
Infectious bursal disease virus, Infectious laryngotracheitis virus, avian
influenza, Newcastle disease virus and fowl pox. Essentially the AGP test
was carried out as described by Woernle (1959). Gels were incubated for 24
hours at 37°C.

When both the IFT and AGP test failed to confirm the identity of the
isolate, IBV antiserum was used to inhibit the potency of the virus infected
allantoic fluid to induce embryo mortality or embryo changes. Initially
only antiserum against the H-vaccine type was used. Later antisera against
this and the four novel serotypes described in this paper were available.
The hyperimmune sera were mixed in equal volumes and the mixture diluted
1:20 with phosphate buffered saline (PBS). Of this mixture 9 volumes were
mixed with 1 volume allantoic fluid and incubated for 30 mins at 40°C
before injection into embryos as before.

PROGRAMME FOR THE CONTROL OF IB

The investigations performed to diminish IBV infections in the
Netherlands can be summarized in the following design:

Stage 1 - Inventory of the incidence of IBV infections

      a. Clinical signs

      b. Serology - AGP

      c. IFT

⇄ Evaluation   a. Low incidence (no further investigations)

                                b. High incidence stage 2

Stage 2 - a. Virus-isolation and serotyping (Cross VN tests)

          b. Serology - check on incidence of antibody against these

                     serotypes in the field (HI; VN)

Stage 3 - Development of vaccines against the predominant serotypes

Stage 4 - Evaluation of the vaccination programme by monitoring flocks

      a. Clinical signs

      b. Serology (seroresponse)

      c. Problem flocks

Be aware of novel serotypes

      stage 2

RESULTS

Stage 1

    A. An example of a flock with egg production problems due to IBV is given in text figure 2. In the figure the precentage of sera from 24 birds reacting positively in the AGP is also expressed. The AGP-curve is in strict harmony with the overall depressed production and with the drop in egg production later on.

    B. Results of the IB diagnosis by IFT in the period 1974-1983 are presented in text figure 3. As demonstrated in the figure outbreaks of IB were observed regularly in 1974. Therefore an investigation was started to devise a better programme for IB vaccination of broilers. As a result of this study, vaccination of day-old chicks in the hatchery was introduced, resulting in a sharp decrease in IB problems. During 1976-1977 IB was diagnosed frequently in laying hens. Vaccination with the H52 vaccine by eye drop resulted in a low incidence of egg problems in breeders and layers in 1978-1979. However in 1980 there was an increase in IB problems in laying hens with dramatically decreased egg production in conjunction with typical

109

TEXT FIGURE 2

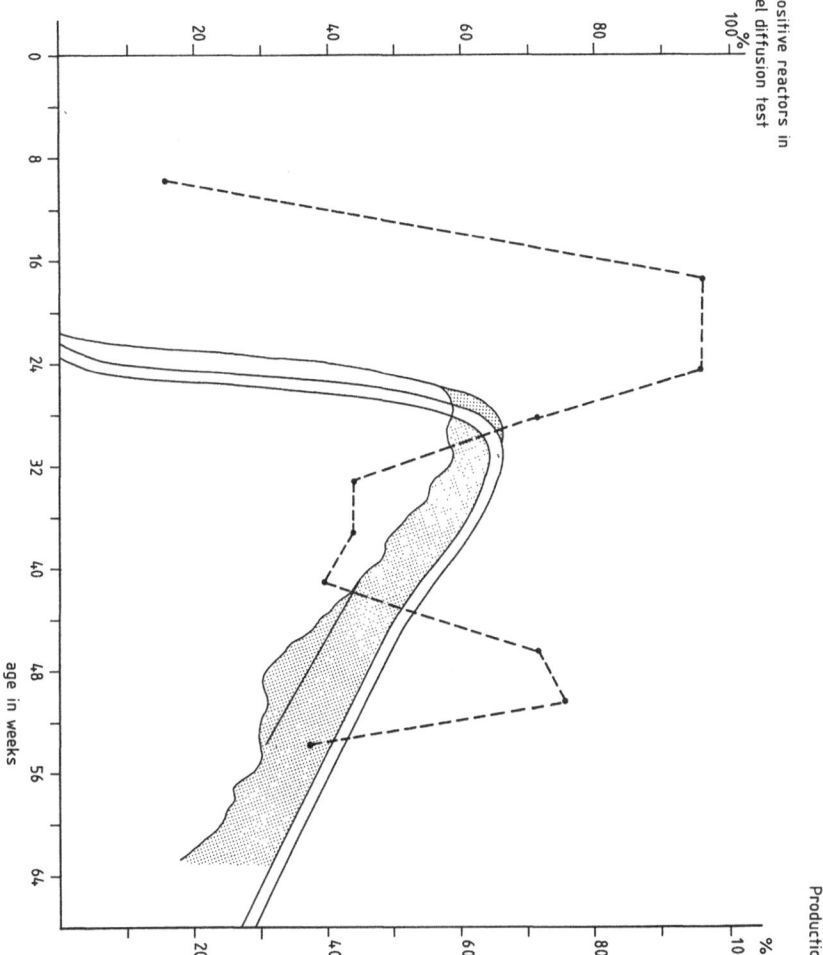

110

TEXT FIGURE 3

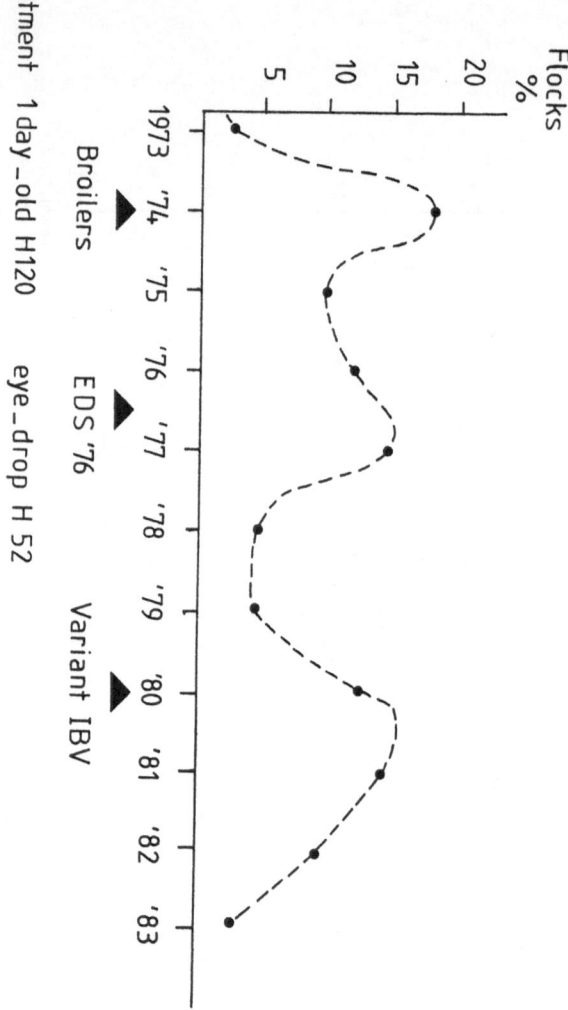

TABLE 2   Survey of IBV isolation trials of 992 flocks suspected of Infectious Bronchitis.

Year	Isolations	D207 No.	D207 %	D212 No.	D212 %	D274 No.	D274 %	Serology D3128 No.	D3128 %	D3896 No.	D3896 %	H52 No.	H52 %	Other No.	Other %
1979	39/167*	19/ 30**	63	4/13	13	-	-	-	-	14/ 31	45	7/ 33	21	2/ 33	6
1980	48/302	13/ 26	50	2/26	8	12/20	60	5/21	24	12/ 26	46	4/ 26	15	1/ 26	4
1981	34/285	6/ 29	21	6/29	21	9/29	31	7/29	24	5/ 29	17	11/ 29	38	1/ 29	3
1982	41/328	2/ 17	12	1/17	6	3/17	18	6/27	35	1/ 17	6	13/ 17	76	2/ 17	12
Total	162/992	40/102	39	13/85	15	24/66	36	18/67	27	32/103	31	35/105	33	6/105	6

* numbers of isolates / numbers of trials to isolate IBV
** number of isolates corresponding with this serotype / number of isolates tested

TABLE 3 Reciprocal cross neutralization test of American strains, Holland 52 Massachusetts type strain and primary IBV isolation of 1978 and 1979.

Virus / serum	I 97	I 609	Connecticut	Florida	JMK	3896	207	212	H52 (Mass.)	3128
I 97	≥6.2	0.7	1.2	1.4	0.7	1.7	0.0	0.0	0.7	1.9
I 609	≤2.9	4.9	≤2.9	≤2.9	≤2.9	3.6	≤2.9	0.0	5.1	≤3.1
Connecticut	2.1	2.1	≥6.8	6.1	1.8	3.6	1.6	≤2.9	4.1	≤2.6
Florida	0.6	1.3	3.4	≥4.2	0.5	2.6	1.0	≤1.2	1.3	4.5
JMK	2.8	1.5	1.4	2.3	≥6.3	2.8	1.3	0.0	1.2	4.5
D3896	≤0.8	0.9	1.5	1.5	≤0.8	≥6.6	1.9	≤0.3	≤0.7	3.2
D207	0.5	0.0	0.4	0.5	≤0.3	2.6	≥5.3	1.3	1.4	3.2
D212	0.0	1.2	1.0	1.0	0.3	2.3	0.5	5.3	0.5	1.4
H52	1.6	2.8	1.8	2.8	1.1	1.8	1.1	1.1	≥5.3	3.7
D274	2.2	2.7	1.9	3.7	2.0	4.2	5.0	≥4.9	≤5.3	3.4
D1466	ND	ND	ND	ND	ND	1.8	1.2	≤1.5	≥1.6	3.1
D3128	1.1	2.1	2.8	3.3	1.3	1.5	0.0	0.0	0.5	≥6.4
D752	1.7	1.7	3.0	1.2	1.9	1.9	1.5	1.3	1.5	1.9

ND = not done

egg shell problems. In most cases IB virus could be demonstrated in the
trachea by means of the IFT. In 1982 and 1983 there was a striking decrease
in the incidence of IB. This was effected by a radical change in the IB
vaccination programs of laying and breeder flocks (see later).

Stage 2

A. Virus isolation and identification. IBV was isolated from 162 of
992 IB suspected flocks during the period 1979–1982 (Davelaar, 1984). This
means that about 16 per cent of the isolation attempts were successful(Table 2). In reciprocal cross–neutralization tests with the American strains
Iowa 97, Iowa 609, Connecticut, Florida, JMK and the Massachusetts type vaccine strain H52, the majority of the primary isolates could be classified
into 4 major serogroups that differ from the American strains and the H52
strain (Table 3). The new serogroups are called D207, D212, D3896 and
D3128 (D = Doorn, the number stands for the laboratory number of the first
isolate). Notice that isolate D274 is closely related to the serogroups
D207 and D3896 (Table 3). Based on the definition that strains with NI values ≥ 4 in cross–neutralization tests with known antisera are considered to
belong to the same serogroup, isolate D274 is classified in both serogroups
D207 and D3896. Further investigations showed that a majority of isolates
corresponding to isolate D274 (NI ≥ 4) are also related with the serogroups
D207 and D3896. Table 2 shows a survey of isolates obtained and characterized during the years 1979–1982. In the years 1979 and 1980 viruses of the
serotypes D207 and D3896 were predominant, thereafter the number of isolates
of these serotypes decreased in favour of the Massachusetts type viruses.

B. Serological survey. The results of a survey of 328 flocks for the
presence of antibody against the IBV serotypes D207, D212, D3896 and D3128
are listed in Table 4. This survey shows a distribution of antibody in

TABLE 4 Frequency of IBV variant types in The Netherlands.
Serological examination of 328 flocks.

Strain (type)	D207	D212	D3128	D3896
Flocks monitored				
No. 328	214	107	180	218
Percentage	65	33	55	66

flocks comparable with the isolation pattern. Antibody to the serotypes

TABLE 5 Ten groups of 12 weeks old chicks (each group 5 birds) were eye drop vaccinated with H120 vaccine strain and challenged by the same route 4 weeks later.

Experimental design			Histology of the trachea				Virus recovery
Group	Vaccinated with H120	Challenge	pre chall.	4 days after	total lesion score	10 days after	4 days after chall.
1.	no	D387		1.8*	1.0*	1.4**	3/5***
2.	no	D207		1.7	1.2	1.4	4/5
3.	no	D212	0*	1.0	0.3	0.7	3/5
4.	no	D3128		2	1.0	1.5	3/5
5.	no	D2896		1.5	1.0	1.3	3/5
6.	yes	D387		0	0.2	0.1	0/5
7.	yes	D207		0.5	0.7	0.6	3/5
8.	yes	D212	0	0.3	0.3	0.3	2/5
9.	yes	D3128		1	0.5	0.8	2/5
10.	yes	D3896		0.9	0.8	0.8	1/5

* Mean lesion score of 6 tracheas per group

** Mean lesion score of 12 tracheas per group collected at 4 and 10 days after challenge

*** Number of embryonated eggs showing abnormalities typical for IBV / number of eggs inoculated with tracheal scrapings.

D207, D3896 and D3128 was observed in 55-66 per cent of the flocks, while antibodies against serotype D212 were present in only 33 per cent of the flocks.

Stage 3

A. Cross-immunity tests in chicks. Cross-immunity tests in chicks were carried out to examine whether vaccination with a Massachusetts type vaccine (H120) would provide protection against the novel serotypes. The results of a challenge experiment are summarized in Table 5. Vaccination with H120 protected the birds against tracheal lesions caused by the Massachusetts type challenge virus (D387), but was not able to reduce the lesions caused by the other strains for more than 50 per cent. The results of the virus recovery test confirmed the histological findings.VI was negative only in group 6, vaccinated with H120 and challenged with Massachusetts type virus. In contrast VI was positive in the H120 vaccinated groups challenged with heterologous viruses and in the non vaccinated challenged chicks. It appears from the lesion scores in Table 5 that the isolates D207, D3896, D3128 and D387 have similar pathogenic properties to the trachea, while the pathogenic effect of isolate D212 is much more limited.

B. Table 6 illustrates the various approaches to control IB by vaccination. We focussed our activities primarily on the search for a virus strain with good immunogenic properties and a broad spectrum. The isolate D274 belonging to the serotype D207 induced cross-protection against D207, D3896 and to a lesser extent against D3128, but no protection against D212 challenge. During further investigation of that vaccine candidate strain, D274, we found out that D274 virus agglutinated chicken red blood cells spontaneously. The agglutination was observed with virus preparations consisting of untreated allantoic fluid harvested 24-72 hours p.i. and with supernatant from infected CEK cell cultures.

TABLE 6 Control of IB by vaccination

Monovalent live vaccine	→	Preferably broad spectrum strains H-strains; strain D274
Polyvalent live vaccine	→	Risk of interference
Inactivated vaccine	→	Polyvalent; use restricted to breeders and layers

SPF birds vaccinated with attenuated (by embryo passage) D274 strains responded with extremely high HI and neutralization antibody titers. The haemagglutinating (HA^+) strain of D274 appeared to be more immunogenic than the non haemagglutinating (HA^-) strains belonging to the same serotype (e. g. isolate D207) (Table 7) (Davelaar, 1983). This observation was confirmed by a series of laboratory experiments which encouraged us to use D274 as a vaccine strain in the field. Spontaneously haemagglutinating strains have since been found among other serotypes and we have some experimental evidence that the immunizing potency of IBV strains showing spontaneous haemagglutination of chicken red blood cells, exceeds the potency of virus strains belonging to the same respective serotypes but which do not spontaneously agglutinate RBC's. Chickens were vaccinated with 10^5 EID_{50} per bird

TABLE 7 Mean HI titer of ten vaccinated hens per group.
HI antigen prepared with IBV D274.

Vaccine	Weeks after vaccination											
	0	1	2	3	4	6	7	8	9	10	11	12
207 (HA^-)	4.0	5.4	6.2	5.9	6.6	4.8	4.2	5.5	5.8	5.2	4.1	5.2
274 (HA^+)	4.7	7.5	8.2	8.7	8.2	10.0	9.3	10.0	10.1	9.5	8.8	9.3
none				←		< 5		→				

by eye drop with experimental vaccines prepared from the HA^- strains D207 and the HA^+ strains D274 respectively. HI antibody response was measured in weekly intervals, the sera were tested for VN AB's at 3 and 12 weeks p. v. and the birds were subjected to a challenge infection with a low egg passage D207 strain 12 weeks p.v. Table 7 shows results of HI testing, peak mean titer 6.6 ↔ 10.0 and 12 weeks p.v. still 9 ↔ 5 in the D207 group. Table 8 demonstrates that the VN response was better in the D274 group 12 weeks p.v.: 9/10 birds had a specific protective titer, 5/10 in the D207 group. The same applies for challenge: complete protection in D274 group- 60% in D207 group against the homologous challenge virus (Table 9). Table 10 illustrates that after combination of two HA^+ strains the immune response is significantly better than in a combined live vaccine consisting of two HA^- strains.

Stage 4
A. Since 1982 we have been working in the field with vaccination pro-

TABLE 8 *Number of animals (out of ten vaccinated) showing a neutralizing response > 4.0 log against the homologous strains

Weeks after vaccination	Vaccine group	
	207 (HA$^-$)	274 (HA$^+$)
3	7/10*	9/10*
12	5/10	9/10

TABLE 9 *Number of birds (out of ten vaccinated) showing microscopical
lesions or positive IFT reactions in the trachea 4 days
after challenge infection.

Vaccine	Microscopic lesions	IFT positive
207 (HA$^-$)	6/10*	2/10
274 (HA$^+$)	0/10	0/10
non	10/10	6/10

grammes based on live IB vaccines (Table 11) alone or in combination with
inactivated vaccines (Table 12). Using these vaccination programmes based
on HA$^+$ isolates the incidence of IB decreased from approximately 12 per
cent to less than 4 per cent within a period of 2 years (text figure 3).
The strains used for these vaccinations and their relation to the Dutch serotypes are expressed in Table 13.

B. Problem flocks. IBV is isolated from flocks suffering from IB.
Changes in the pattern of isolations during the period 1980–1985 are presented in Table 14.

TABLE 10 HI response* after vaccination with different live IB
vaccines of D207 serotype.

Vaccine	Mean HI titer of ten birds* weeks after eye drop vaccination				
	0	2	4	6	8
D274 (HA$^+$)	4.0	9.8	10.0	10.0	10.3
D274 + D1466 (HA$^+$)	3.9	8.0	9.0	8.4	9.0
Commercial combined					
D207 + D212 (HA$^-$)	3.9	6.2	6.6	5.2	5.9
Controls	3.8	4.0	3.9	3.6	4.2

*HI test against serotype D207

TABLE 11   Vaccination program of laying and breeder flocks based on live vaccines

1 day	Mareks disease	Injection at hatchery
1 day	IB, H120	Spray at hatchery
1 week	ND, H or C	Knap sack
2-3 weeks	Gumboro disease	Drinking water
5 weeks	ND, H C or L	Knap sack or Atomist
8-10 weeks	IB, D1466	Eye drop or knap sack
10-12 weeks	IB, D274	Knap sack (or eye drop)
12-14 weeks	Epidemic tremor	Oral or spray or drinking water
	ILT	Eye drop
	Fowl pox	Wing web
14-16 weeks	IB, H52	Eye drop or knap sack
16-20 weeks	ND, C or L	Atomist

```
ND  = Newcastle disease
H   = Hitchner
C   = Clone 30 (Intervet ND vaccines)
L   = LaSota strain of ND
ILT = Infectious Laryno Tracheitis
```

TABLE 12   Vaccination program for laying and breeder flocks based on live and inactivated vaccines.

1 day	Mareks disease	Injection at hatchery
1 day	IB, H120	Spray at hatchery
1 week	ND, H or C	Knap sack
2-3 weeks	Gumboro disease	Drinking water
5 weeks	ND, H, C or L	Knap sack or Atomist
8-10 weeks	IB, D1466	Eye drop or knap sack
10-12 weeks	IB, D274	Knap sack (or eye drop)
12-14 weeks	Epidemic tremor	Oral or spray or drinking water
	ILT	Eye drop
	Fowl pox	Wing web
16-20 weeks	IB, H' + variant strains	Injection
	ND	Injection
	Gumboro disease	Injection reproduction
	EDS	Injection, infected farms

```
Explanation see Table 11
Variant strains = D274 + D1466
H'              = Massachusetts type strain M41
EDS             = Egg drop syndrome
```

In 1980-1982 about 90 per cent of the isolates (79) were classified into one of the 4 serogroups (NI ≥4). In contrast in 1984-1985 37 per cent of the isolates (110) did not belong to one of these serogroups. They showed

TABLE 13 IBV serotype, their HI antigens and vaccine strains.

Serotype	Mass.	D207	D3895	D3128	D212
HI-antigen	M41	D274 (HA$^+$)			D1466 (HA$^+$)
Vaccine strains	H120 H52 M41	D274 (HA$^+$)			D1466 (HA$^+$)

weak to moderate cross-reactions with the serotypes D1466, D3128 and H52. This suggests that the highly immunogenic vaccine strain D274 prevents mutation of viruses of the same serotype. Other less immunogenic vaccines (H120; H52 and D1466) may permit mutation (shift and drift). Although IB problems have decreased at the moment, it is necessary to keep the situation in the field under close surveillance. The findings mentioned above indicate the risk of the development of IB viruses which cannot be controlled with the available vaccines.

REFERENCES

Alexander, D.J. and Chettle, N.J. 1977. Procedures for the haemagglutination inhibition tests for avian infectious bronchitis virus. Avian Pathology, 6, 9.
Bijlenga, G. 1975. Het infektieuze bronchitis virus bij kuikens in Nederland aangetoond met behulp van ei-enting, dierexperimenteel onderzoek en serumneutralizatieproeven. Tijdschrift voor Diergeneeskunde, 81, 43.
Davelaar, F.G., Noordzij, A. and Donk, J.A. van der, 1982. A study on the synthesis and secretion of immunoglobulins by the Harderian gland of the fowl after eye drop vaccination against infectious bronchitis at one-day-old. Avian Pathology, 11, 63.
Davelaar, F.G., Kouwenhoven, B., Burger, A.G. and Lutticken, D. 1983. Signification des Serotypes variants de la brochite inf. aviaire aux Pays-Bas. L'aviculteur, 436,5.
Davelaar, F.G., Kouwenhoven, B. and Burger,A.G. 1984. Occurrence and significance of Infectious Bronchitis variant strains in egg and broiler production in the Netherlands. The Veterinary Quarterly, 6, 144.
Jaspers, D, Hemmes, W. Weststrate, M.W. and Davelaar, F.G. 1984. The use of live and inactivated infectious bronchitis vaccines including Massachusetts and IB-variant serotypes in broiler-breeder and commercial layer flocks. Proceedings XVII World's Poultry Congress, Helsinki.
Kouwenhoven, B., Davelaar, F.G., Burger, A.G. and Lutticken, D. 1983. Significance of variant IB serotypes in the Netherlands. Australian Veterinary Poultry Association; the international union of immunological societies - proceedings no. 66, 53.
Lukert, P.D. 1975. Infectious bronchitis. In: Isolation and identification of avian pathogens. Hitchner, S.B., Domermuth, C.H., Purchase, H.G. and Williams, J.E. eds. pp 182 Am. Assoc. Avian Pathologists.

120

TABLE 14

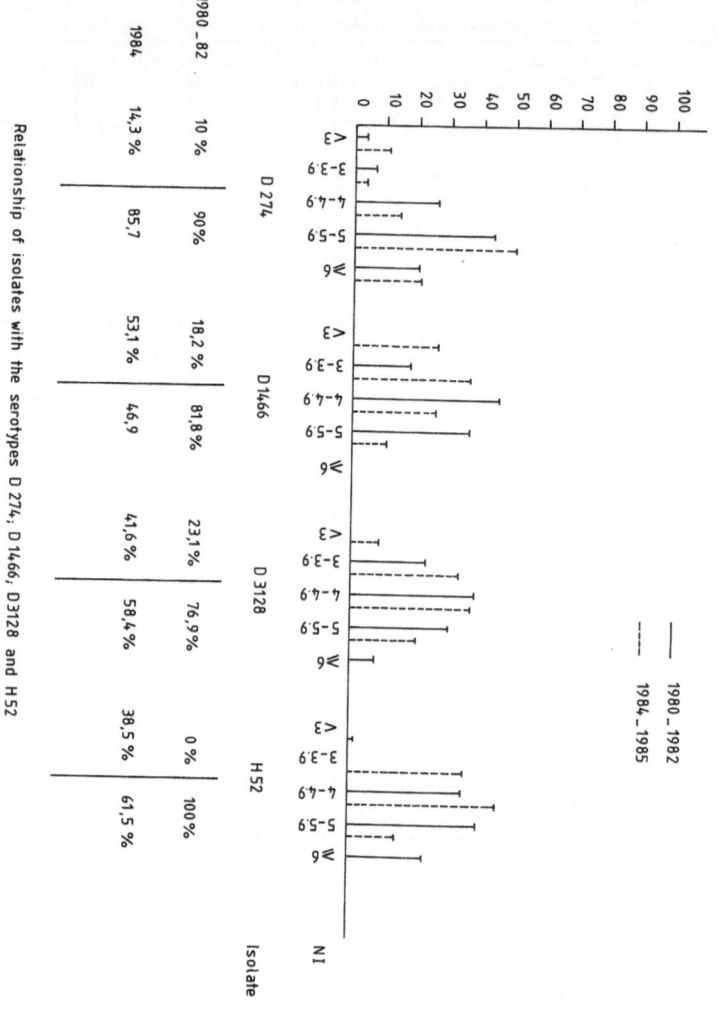

	D 274		D 1466		D 3128		H 52	
1980 - 82	10 %	90%	18,2 %	81,8%	23,1 %	76,9%	0 %	100%
1984	14,3 %	85,7	53,1 %	46,9	41,6 %	58,4%	38,5 %	61,5 %

—— 1980 - 1982
– – – 1984 - 1985

Relationship of isolates with the serotypes D 274; D 1466; D 3128 and H 52

Winterfield, R.W. and Fadly, M.A. 1975. Potential for polyvalent infectious bronchitis vaccines. American Journal of Veterinary Research,
  36, 524.
Woernle, H. 1959. Diagnose der Infektiosen Bronchitis der Huhner mit
  Hilfe der prazipitations Reaktion im festen Agar Medium. Monatshefte
  fur Tierheilkunde, 11, 154.

A NEW PATHOGENIC AVIAN INFECTIOUS BRONCHITIS VIRUS ISOLATED IN FRANCE

J.P. Picault*, G. Bennejean*, P. Drouin*, M. Guittet*, J. Protais*,

R. L'Hospitalier*, J. P. Gillet**,

J. Lamande*, A. Le Bachelier*

Ministere de L'Agriculture, Direction de la Qualité, Services Vétérinaires
*   Laboratoire National de Pathologie Aviaire et Station Experimen-
tale d'Aviculture, B.P. 9, 22440 PLOUFRAGAN, FRANCE
** Laboratoire Central de Recherches Vétérinaires, B.P. 67
94703 MAISONS-ALFORT CEDEX, FRANCE

ABSTRACT

A coronavirus was isolated in an infectious bronchitis (IB) vaccinated
(Massachusetts strain) layer flock showing severe IB-like clinical signs.
The isolate is antigenically different from the Massachusetts and the
Connecticut serotypes and from the four "variant" serotypes isolated by
the Doorn Institute in Holland. The disease was reproduced in chickens
and layers. Respiratory signs were severe in both groups. In layers, egg
drop was intense and long-lasting. The eventual development of a suitable
medical prophylaxy is discussed.

INTRODUCTION

Infectious bronchitis (IB) is one of the main diseases of the fowl.
Vaccines prepared using only the Massachusetts (Mass) serotype are used in
France to prevent the disease. Some failures were initially attributed to
vaccination procedures. However from 1976 to 1981 several authors (Jones,
1976; Meulemans et al., 1976; Davelaar et al., 1981; Cook, 1983) have
isolated and characterized "variant" coronaviruses (IBVV) in IB-like field
cases in Europe. Some of these give a poor cross-protection with Mass-
vaccines.

This paper describes isolation and characterization of a coronavirus
with interesting antigenic and pathogenic properties. This virus has been
called PL-84084 (Ploufragan; LNPA; 1984; sample number 084).

CLINICAL STUDY OF THE FIELD CASE

The PL-84084 virus was isolated in Brittany in February 1984, in a
41 week old 6100 laying hens flock. These conventional birds had been
routinely vaccinated during the rearing period against several diseases
and particularly against IB as follows : H120 live vaccine by spray at day
old and four weeks old, and Mass-inactivated oil adjuvant vaccine by injection at 19 weeks of age.

At 40 weeks old, birds showed respiratory distress with an extended neck during inspiration and tracheal rales. There was no obvious nasal discharge or diarrhea. All birds were affected but additional mortality did not exceed 2.6% between 40 and 44 weeks of age. Dead birds presented a purplish-blue comb, a catarrhal cloacitis, a tracheitis with catarrhal inflammation, pin point haemorrhages and muco-purulent exudate, congested and hypertrophied kidneys, and sometimes congested and flaccid ovules and a catarrhal inflammation of the vagina. Purulent salpingitis and intra-abdominal laying were observed between 44 and 48 weeks of age.

There was a slight decrease in food consumption and a fall in egg production of four weeks duration with a maximum production loss of 14%. At the same time the egg weight was 1.5g less than previously. Shell discoloration and a marked increase in the proportion of weak shelled eggs were observed.

ETIOLOGICAL STUDY

Virus isolation and serological diagnosis

Virus isolation was performed in SPF hens' eggs inoculated with the supernatant of tracheal and lung homogenates from hens showing signs for approximately three days. During the third blind passage, embryo mortality occurred at three days P.I. Dead and surviving embryos showed lesions typical of coronavirus infection. Investigations to detect other agents possibly involved in the disease notably myxoviruses and infectious laryngo-tracheitis virus, were negative.

A precipitating antigen was prepared from the chorioallantoic membranes of dead eggs. A positive agar gel precipitation (AGP) was obtained by using this antigen and a monospecific-hyperimmune Massachusetts antiserum. Cross AGP reactions showed a common precipitating line with Mass.

Allantoic fluids from dead eggs contained typical coronavirus particles when observed with an electron microscope after negative staining with phosphotungstic acid.

Coronaviral seroconversion of convalescent hens was clearly demonstrated, due to the presence in the infected house of white Leghorn SPF laying hens habitually introduced as sentinels with the conventional layers at the beginning of lay. These SPF layers had little or no coronavirus antibodies at the time of the first respiratory signs. Two weeks later, they showed Beaudette AGP antibodies (19/19 positive) and Mass haemagglutination inhibiting antibodies ($2^{6.6}$ mean titre). Ten weeks after the signs, when tested for neutralising antibodies using the alpha method, they showed PL-84084 antibodies (index $>$ 6.11), but no significant Beaudette antibodies (index $<$ 3.07).

Determination of PL-84084 serotype

A specific PL-84084 antiserum was prepared in White Leghorn SPF chickens, to be used in cross alpha seroneutralisation tests against our available IB coronaviruses : Beaudette, Connecticut, and six Dutch IB-variant strains kindly provided by Drs Davelaar and Kouwenhoven from the Doorn Institute in the Netherlands, i.e D-207, D-212, D-3128, D-3896, D-274 and D-1466.

All virus titres were pre-adjusted between $10^{6.5}$ and 10^{7} EID 50 per ml before sequential tenfold dilutions in PBS.

Sera were pre-diluted to 1/25. 0.4 ml of each virus dilution was added to the same volume of prediluted sera and incubated at room temperature for 30 minutes. Then 0.1 ml of each mixture was inoculated into each of 5 nine day old embryonated SPF eggs. The eggs were incubated for nine days at 37°C and candled daily. Embryos dying within 24 hours after inoculation were discarded. Other dead embryos and the remaining live ones at the end of the experimental period were examined for lesions. The end point titre for each serum/virus mixture was calculated by the method of Reed and Muench for the determination of the neutralisation index. Results are given in Table 1. They reveal antigenic difference between strain PL-84084 and the eight other strains tested. With some Dutch serotypes the differences between homologous and heterologous index were not high, probably due to low sera titres.

TABLE 1.   Cross-seroneutralisation indices.

Virus or Serum "x"	Homologous reaction	Heterologous reaction	
		Virus PL-84084 + Serum "x"	Virus "x" + serum PL-84084
PL-84084	$>$ 5.28	–	–
Massachusetts	$>$ 5.12	$<$ 1.81	$<$ 2.42
Connecticut	4.07	1.41	1.90
D-207	4.55	2.22	2.89
D-212	$>$ 5.27	1.40	1.68
D-3128	4.31	2.56	1.40
D-3896	5.70	2.40	2.65
D-274	5.37	2.79	3.12
D-1466	6.40	2.39	2.80

EXPERIMENTAL REPRODUCTION OF THE DISEASE

In SPF chicks

30 day old and 30 fifteen day old White Leghorn SPF chicks were inoculated by eye drop with $10^{3.3}$ EID 50 of strain PL-84084. Clinical signs
were recorded daily during a four week-long period after inoculation. Individual respiratory signs were classified on a scale from 0 to 4, depending on their intensity. A score of 4 was attributed to birds with a very
severe respiratory distress or/and mortality. An average score was calculated, taking account of all birds into the group, and not only the sick
birds.

From the third day P.I, about 80% of birds in both groups showed
tracheo-bronchitis signs, with some showing severe respiratory distress.
Average intensity of respiratory signs was scored 2.5 in the day old group,
as against 2.0 in the fifteen day old group. Duration of individual respiratory signs was 22 days in the first group as against only 7 days in
the second. Neither nasal discharge, diarrhea, nor mortality were observed. Classical macroscopic and microscopic lesions of IB were seen. The
most severely affected organs were the trachea, lungs and Harderian gland
in both groups, and in addition, the kidneys and liver in two of the
youngest birds.

In conventional layers

96 White Leghorn hens were conventionally reared from day old to 21
weeks of age. They were vaccinated against several diseases, and notably
against IB with live H120 vaccine administered by spray at day old, 4 and
12 weeks of age. At 21 weeks of age, they were divided into three groups
housed separately. Two groups (group RC, and half the birds in group R)
were revaccinated with a Mass-inactivated oil adjuvanted vaccine (IOAV).
Just after peak of lay, at 28 weeks of age, a revaccinated group (RC) and
the unrevaccinated group (C) were challenged by spray with strain PL-84084
(Table 2).

Respiratory signs were registered and scored daily from 0 to 4 as before. Egg production and egg quality were recorded weekly before challenge
and for 13 weeks after challenge. A gross autopsy was carried out in birds
dying during the observation period and in a sample of birds per group at
slaughtering.

TABLE 2. Experimental design.

Group	No of layers	IB Vaccinations		PL-84084 challenge
		Live H 120	Mass-IOAV	
R	32	1 D, 4 and 12 W	21 W (16 birds)	—
C	32	1 D, 4 and 12 W	—	28 W
RC	32	1 D, 4 and 12 W	21 W	28 W

Control birds (R) showed neither respiratory signs, egg-drop,abnormal eggs nor specific macroscopic lesions during the observation period. The challenged birds (groups C and RC) presented severe respiratory signs, beginning three days P.I. but lasting no more than five days. The average intensity of these signs was 3.8 in group C and 3.2 in group RC. One to two weeks after challenge, both groups showed a marked egg drop, of 42% in group C and 26% in group RC. During the 13 weeks observation period, normal egg production was below predicted production levels by about 27% in group C and 20% in group RC. As White Leghorn hens produce white eggs, shell discoloration was not observed. This probably explains why abnormal eggs were not seen earlier than four weeks P.I. Abnormalities were typical of IB i.e., shell-less, soft-shelled, thin-shelled, misshapen or small eggs. Production of such eggs reached a maximum of 25% in group C and 16% in group RC. Numerous bloody stained normal shelled eggs were observed in the challenged groups only but they were not considered as abnormal eggs.

In addition to respiratory signs and egg drop, hens from challenged groups showed diarrhoea throughout the observation period. Macroscopic lesions observed in birds dying during the trial and in birds slaughtered at the end of the experiment were confined to the reproductive tract. The absence of respiratory tract lesions was probably due to too long a delay between respiratory signs and necropsy. Genital lesions consisted of cloacitis, partial occlusion of ovary and vagina, salpingitis and caseous nodules in the oviduct.

DISCUSSION - CONCLUSION

As a serological survey conducted in French poultry farms two years ago had revealed the infection of numerous flocks with coronaviruses belonging to the Dutch IB variant serotypes, but failed to establish a correlation between the presence of these IBVV-antibodies and IB-like clinical signs (Picault et al., 1984), it was necessary to try to isolate such variant viruses in severe outbreaks. The first one,PL-84084,proved to be antigenically different from not only Mass and Connecticut but also from the Dutch serotypes. The pathogenic properties of this strain were demonstrated both in chickens and in laying hens, as was the insufficient protection conferred by a Mass vaccination program in layers. It could be said that our challenge was too severe but we perform the same challenge procedure to control the potency of Mass-IOAV, and generally obtain good protection against challenge with Mass 41. Furthermore we now have evidence that strain PL-84084 was involved in a second outbreak in layers revaccinated at beginning of lay with a Mass-IOAV. It remains to be seen whether Dutch IB variant vaccines could give a significant cross protection against our viral strain. We are also beginning an epidemiological survey in order to detect other PL-84084 outbreaks. Whatever the results of this survey may be, the isolation of a strain like PL-84084 confirms the necessity of a continuous surveillance of the IB situation, as suggested by others (Davelaar et al., 1981; Cook, 1984).

REFERENCES

Cook, J.K.A. 1983. Isolation of a new serotype of infectious bronchitis-like virus from chickens in England. The Veterinary Record, 112, 104-105.
Cook, J.K.A. 1984. The classification of new serotypes of infectious bronchitis virus isolated from poultry flocks in Britain between 1981 and 1983. Avian Pathology, 13, 733-741.
Davelaar, F.G., Kouwenhoven, B. and Burger, A.G. 1981. Investigations into the significance of infectious bronchitis virus (IBV) variant strains in broiler and egg production. Proceedings of World Veterinary Poultry Association, Oslo, 1981, p.44.
Jones, R.C. 1976. The isolation and some biological properties of a variant infectious bronchitis virus. The Veterinary Record, 98, 278-279.
Meulemans, G., Vindevogel, H., Burtonboy, G., Deylgat, A. and Halen, P. 1976. Isolement d'un nouveau sérotype du virus de la bronchite infectieuse aviaire en Belgique. Annales de Médecine Vétérinaire, 120, 199-204.
Picault, J.P., Bennejean, G., Guittet, M., Le Jeune, M., Le Coq, H. and Le Bachelier, A. 1984. Enquête sérologique concernant les virus "variants" de la bronchite infectieuse aviaire (BI) en France. Actes et abstraits du XVIIème Congrès Mondial d'Aviculture organisé par la W.P.S.A. à Helsinki, 1984, 527-529.

ANTIGENIC DIFFERENTIATION OF AVIAN BRONCHITIS VIRUS VARIANT STRAINS EMPLOYING MONOCLONAL ANTIBODIES

G. Koch, L. Hartog, A. Kant, D. van Roozelaar and G.F. de Boer

Central Veterinary Institute, Dept. of Virology,
Postbox 365, 8200 AJ Lelystad, The Netherlands.

ABSTRACT

Monoclonal antibodies (McAbs) to Infectious Bronchitis Virus (IBV) were prepared and tested for reactivity to different IBV variant strains by an indirect enzyme-immunoassay.

With the exception of two McAbs specific for the nucleoprotein, which did not recognize the SE-17 strain, all McAbs to the matrix and nucleoprotein reacted with all strains tested. McAbs to the matrix and nucleoprotein, therefore, are suitable for diagnostic purposes.

On basis of the reactivity pattern to variant strains of a panel of McAbs specific for the peplomer protein, it was possible to differentiate Dutch variant strains into three groups .

INTRODUCTION

Infectious Bronchitis is a highly contagious, mainly respiratory disease of young chickens. The disease is of economical importance because infection of production flocks and broilers often leads to permanent decrease in egg-laying and growth retardation, respectively. The causative agent is a virus, Infectious Bronchitis Virus (IBV), which belongs to the family of the Coronaviridae.

Although there have been much disagreement on the actual number of IBV structural proteins in the past, it is now generally accepted that IBV contains three structural proteins only (Cavanagh, 1981; Stern et al. 1982; Stern and Sefton 1982). The three structural proteins are a non-glycosylated nucleoprotein (N), and two glycosylated envelope proteins. The nucleoprotein is a phosphorylated protein (Lomniczi and Morser, 1981) with a molecular weight of 50 to 55 kdalton. In the virus particle, N is complexed to a genomic RNA molecule. Together they form the nucleocapsid of the virus. The matrix of the virus consists mainly of a trans-membrane protein (M) embedded in a lipid layer. M is an heterogenous glycoprotein with a molecular weight ranging from 23 to 36 kdalton depending on the extent of glycosylation. The surface protein, which in the electron microscope has a morphology of a peplomer, contains two non-covalently linked subunits S1 and S2. S1 and S2 have molecular weights of 92 and 84 kdalton, respectively. Based on experimental evidence of Cavanagh (1983a, 1983b), it is concluded that S2 subunits form the stick, whereas S1 subunits form the bulb of the peplomer.

The control of IB still is difficult and tedious with outbreaks of the disease occurring both in vaccinated and unvaccinated flocks. Vaccination breaks are attributed, in part, to new antigenically distinct strains. Since the start of the vaccination programme in the Netherlands two decades ago, a large number of new isolates have been obtained and characterized. These isolates are classified into four antigenically distinct groups by serum neutralization (SN) and haem-agglutination inhibition (HI) tests (Locker et al., 1983; Cook, 1984; Davelaar et al. 1984). Both tests, however, show different levels of cross-reactivity patterns of individual sera to heterologous variant strains. Furthermore, in the SN test different results are often obtained when different indicator systems for virus infectivity are used (Cowen and Hitchner, 1975). As a consequence, tests performed at a different time or place often result in different antigenic groupings. New IBV isolates are initially difficult to propagate in the usual in vitro cell culture systems (Sturman and Holmes, 1983; Hofstad, 1984) and the serological characterization by SN and HI tests needs the preparation of homologous antisera. Furthermore, the characterization is hampered by the numerous, but ill defined, antigenic groupings proposed. Therefore, diagnosis and characterization of new field strains is time consuming.

Monoclonal antibodies (McAbs) are continuously produced by immortal hybrid cell lines obtained by the deliberate fusion of myeloma cells and B lymphocytes. Since cloned hybrid cell lines are derived from single B lymphocytes, these cell lines provide us with a source of highly specific antibodies in unlimited quantities. In this way antibodies with specificity for distinct epitopes of different proteins can be obtained.

McAbs to structural proteins of IBV could provide us with techniques for rapid diagnosis and antigenic characterization of IBV isolates in a more simple fashion. For this reason, and to map the antigenic relationships of IBV variant strains at the epitope level, which could provide valuable information useful for the formulation of new vaccines, we prepared McAbs to the three structural proteins of IBV. This report gives an overview of the results obtained up to now.

MATERIALS AND METHODS

Viruses

The IBV variant strains were originally obtained from Laboratory Dr. de Zeeuw, De Bilt, The Netherlands (0728, B801, U101, G901-20 and L502) and from the Poultry Health Service, Doorn, The Netherlands (D207, D274, D3128, D3896,

D212 and D1466). The virus strains were received at different embryonic passages. For the adaptation of the virus to grow in chicken embryo kidney (CEK) cells, the viruses were serially passaged in CEKC monolayers until a cytopathological effect could be observed.

Virus growth and purification

Virus was grown on 11-day-old embryonated eggs. Approximately 10^4 median egg infectious dose of virus was injected into the allantoic cavity. After incubation for 24 hr at $38^{\circ}C$, the eggs were chilled at $4^{\circ}C$ and subsequently the allantoic fluid was harvested. To remove cellular debris the allantoic fluid was centrifuged at 800 g for 30 minutes. Virus was concentrated from the allantoic fluid by centrifugation for about 24 hr at 10,000 g in a Beckman J-21 centrifuge. The virus pellet was resuspended in TSE buffer (0.01 M Tris-hydrochloride, 0.1 M sodium chloride and 1 mM EDTA). Subsequently, the virus was purified by velocity sedimentation overnight at $4^{\circ}C$ through a linear 26 to 65% (w/v) sucrose gradient using a Beckman SW-27 rotor (Cavanagh, 1981). The protein concentration of the virus preparation was determined using bovine serum albumine (BSA) as a standard (Lowry et al., 1951). The virus preparations were stored at $-70^{\circ}C$ until use.

Preparation of monoclonal antibodies

BALB/c mice, 10-14 weeks of age, were primed by an intraperitoneal inoculation of 50 ug purified IBV emulsified in CFA. After 6 to 8 weeks, the mice were boosted intravenously with the same dose of purified IBV. The fusion of immune spleen cells, harvested 3 days after the booster immunization, and the non-secretor plasmacytoma cells, P3-X-63Ag8.653 (Kearny et al., 1979), was performed according to the technique originally described by Kohler and Milstein (1975) with some slight modifications (Van Zaane and IJzerman, 1984). Peritoneal macrophages were used as feeder cells (Fazekas de St. Groth and Scheidegger, 1980).

Screening of the culture fluids for antiviral antibodies was performed with an indirect enzyme-immunoassay (EIA). As control the fluids were tested for reactivity to proteins present in allantoic fluids of uninfected eggs (AF) and to New castle Disease Virus (NCD). Cells, lines which scored positive in the EIA for IBV and negative for AF and NCD, were cloned by limiting dilution combined with visual inspection. Clones were expanded after the third cloning procedure. Ascites fluid was subsequently produced in pristane treated BALB/c mice (Brodeur et al., 1984).

Enzyme-immunoassay

The enzyme-immunoassay (EIA) was performed on antigen-coated polystyrene microtiter plates (Dynatech M129 A, Cooke). The plates were coated overnight at $4^{o}C$ with either 0.5-1 µg purified IBV, the same amount of NCD or 12 µg AF diluted in sodium bicarbonate buffer pH 9.6 per well. The plates were stored at $4^{o}C$ in the same buffer until use. In the antibody binding assay, culture fluid or ascites fluid was serially diluted in EIA diluent (phosphate buffered saline supplemented with 51 gr of sodium chloride per liter, 0.05% Tween 20 and 4% normal horse serum (NHS)) and incubated for 90 minutes at $37^{o}C$, which was the incubation temperature at all subsequent steps as well. Subsequently, the plates were incubated with horse-radish peroxidase conjugated to rabbit anti-mouse immunoglobulin (RAM/Ig-PO) (Nordic Lab., Tilburg, The Netherlands) and, finally, stained in a solution of 1 mg/ml 5-amino-2-benzoic acid (5-aminosalicylic acid) (Merck Chemicals, Darmstadt) in phosphate buffer pH 5.95 to which, prior to use, freshly-prepared H_2O_2 was added to a final concentration of 0.05 per cent. The peroxidase activity was quantified by measuring the optical density at 450 nm in a Titertek Multiscan (Flow).

Microneutralization test

The SN test was performed essentially as described previously (Blore and Skeeles, 1981). In short, a constant amount of virus (between 100-250 median tissue culture infectious dose ($TCID_{50}$) was mixed with two-fold dilutions of antisera and incubated for 1 hr at room temperature. Subsequently, the virus-serum mixtures were transferred to wells of microtiter plates which contained monolayers of primary CEKC. The plates were placed in a CO_2 incubator at $38-39^{o}C$ for 48 hrs. To score for IBV-infected cultures, the monolayers were fixed with paraformal-dehyde solution and stained by incubation with homologous IBV antiserum and subsequently a goat anti-chick Ig peroxidase conjugate, essentially as described before (Saunders, 1977).

RESULTS

A large number of clones producing McAbs to IBV were obtained. All selected clones produced McAbs which reacted positive in the IBV EIA and negative in the EIA of NCD and AF. The viral protein specificity of the McAbs was characterized by immunoblotting. The results, which will be published in greater detail elsewhere, are summarized below. According to their specificity, McAbs fell into three different groups: Those reacting to M, those reacting to N and those reacting to S. McAbs to S were specific for the S2 subunit which was concluded from the comparison of the staining pattern of McAbs to S with the staining pattern of polyclonal homologous chicken antisera to IBV. McAbs which did not bind to any protein in the IBV blots were discarded for the time being.

Neutralizing activity of the McAbs

The neutralizing activity of the McAbs was determined in the SN test on CEKC monolayers. Only McAbs mentioned in Table I possessed neutralizing activity. All these McAbs were specific for the S2 subunit of the peplomer protein. The titers never exceeded 1 in 640, rather low considering the antibody concentration in the ascites fluids. Increased but also decreased titers were observed when mixtures of distinct McAbs were prepared. Particularly, increased

TABLE I. **Neutralizing activity of monoclonal antibodies and mixtures thereof.**

Monoclonal antibody	—	in combination with monoclonal antibody							
		31.1	31.2	31.3	31.4	31.5	31.6	31.7	31.8
31.1	40[a]								
31.2	0	0							
31.3	80	80	40						
31.4	0	0	0	20					
31.5	80	0	0	1280	0				
31.6	320	640	20	1280	320	80			
31.7	320	80	320	2560	40	40	80		
31.8	320	320	n.d.[b]	320	n.d.	n.d.	640	40	
31.5+31.6	80	40	80	640	n.d.	n.d.	n.d.	1280	160
26.1	≤640	n.d.	n.d.	n.d.	n.d.	n.d.	n.d.	n.d.	n.d.
30.6	≤640	n.d.	n.d.	n.d.	n.d.	n.d.	n.d.	n.d.	n.d.

[a] Reciproke of the neutralizing titer of McAb in an *in vitro* micro neutralization test. Twofold serial dilutions of ascites fluid, heat inactivated for 30 min at 56°C, were incubated with a constant amount of IBV (100-250 $TCID_{50}$). Subsequently, the mixtures were plated on CEKC monolayers.
[b] n.d., not done.

titers were observed when McAb 31.3 was mixed with other McAbs (Table 1, first compared to fourth column). The virus was always completely neutralized.

Cross-reactivity of McAbs to IBV variant strains

The cross-reactivity of the McAbs to IBV was tested in an indirect EIA using microtiter plates coated with several different variant strains. The variant strains used in this test are claimed to belong to four Dutch (Locher et al. 1983; Cook, 1984; Davelaar et al. 1984) and seven American serotypes (Cowen, 1971; Hopkins, 1974; Cowen and Hitchner, 1975; Johnson and Marquardt, 1975; Darbyshire et al., 1979; Hofstad, 1981). The protein composition of all virus preparations used were evaluated by immunoblotting of the IBV variant strains with homologous polyvalent antisera to ascertain that no negative reactions would be scored by the EIA, because proteins were lacking in any of the preparations.

TABLE II.   Reactivity pattern of panel of monoclonal antibodies to IBV

Monoclonal antibody	Specificity	Virus strain													
		H120	B222	M41	D207	D274	D3896	D212	D1466	Clarck	Ark	SE-17	Holte	I97	I609
25.1	M[a]	+++[b]	+++	+++	+++	+++	+++	+++	+++	+++	+++	+++	+++	+++	+++
26.2	N	+++	+++	+++	+++	+++	+++	+++	+++	+++	+++	−	+++	+++	+++
26.3		+++	+++	+++	+++	+++	+++	+++	+++	+++	+++	−	+++	+++	+++
26.1		+++	+++	+++	+++	+++	+++	+++	+++	−	++	+++	+	+	−
30.6		+++	+++	+++	+++	+++	++	+	++	−	++	+++	+	+	+
31.3		+++	+++	+++	++	+++	++	+	+++	−	+	++	+	+	+
32.3		+++	+++	+++	+++	+++	++	−	−	+++	++	+++	+	++	+
31.7		+++	+++	+++	+++	+++	+	−	++	−	+	++	−	−	+
31.1	S$_2$	+++	+++	+++	+++	+++	++	−	++	−	++	++	−	−	−
31.5		++	++++	−	−	−	−	−	−	−	−	−	−	−	−
31.4		++	++++	+++	−	−	−	+	++	−	−	−	−	−	−
30.7		−	++	−	+++	++	++	−	−	−	−	−	−	−	−
32.1		−	+++	−	++	+++	+	−	−	−	−	−	−	−	−
32.2		−	−	−	++	+++	+	−	−	−	−	−	−	−	−
32.5		−	−	−	+++	+++	+	−	−	−	−	−	−	−	−
30.2		−	−	−	+++	+++	++	−	−	++	−	−	−	−	−

[a] The specificity of monoclonal antibodies (McAb) was tested with the immuno-electroblotting technique. M = matrix protein, N = nucleoprotein, S$_2$ = subunit of peplomer protein S.

[b] Reactivity of McAb to IBV. The optical density (O.D.) obtained after binding of McAb to heterologous IBV is expressed as a percentage of the maximal O.D. found after binding to homologous virus. +++ > 50%, ++ 25-50%, + twice background-25%, − less than twice background.

The McAbs specific for M (25.1) and N (26.2, 26.3) reacted to all variant strains in the test to the same extent with the exception of the SE-17 strain which was not recognized by both McAbs to N (Table II). McAbs to M and N produced by 20 respectively 3 uncloned hybrid cell lines likewise demonstrated a broad spectrum of reactivity (data not shown).

McAbs directed to S2 showed much less cross-reactivity. Roughly, on basis of the cross-reactivity, the McAbs to S2 could be divided into four groups: Those reacting to most Dutch and American strains, those (31.5) reacting to Massachusetts serotype only, those (31.4) reacting to the Mass. and one Dutch serotype (D212 and D1466 are claimed to belong to the same serotype), and those reacting to more than one Dutch serotype only.

By comparison of the reactivity patterns of McAbs belonging to the first group, differentiation between a number of American variant strains could be made. For instance, comparing the reactivity pattern of McAb 32.3 to the patterns of McAbs 30.6 and 31.3, a distinction between the Clark strain and the rest of the American strains, i.e. Ark, SE-17, Holte, I97 and I609, could be made. Comparison of the reactivity patterns of McAb 26.1 and 30.6 differentiated the I609 strain from the other strains and so on.

Using a panel of four McAbs, each representative of a group, it was possible to differentiate Dutch variant strains into three groups according to the reaction with the panel. The first group consists of the B222 and L502 strains which are recognized by three McAbs of the panel, but not by McAb 30.2. The second group, consisting of the strains D207, D274, D3896, D3128, O728, U201, L536 and G901-20, is recognized by comparing the reactivity patterns of McAbs 32.3 and 31.4. The third group includes the strains D212, D1466, U101, U121 and B801 which reacted with McAb 31.4 but not with any of the other McAbs of the panel (Table III).

TABLE III. Reactivity pattern of panel of monoclonal antibodies to the S_2 protein[a] of IBV

Monoclonal antibody	B222	L502	D207	D274	D3128	D3896	O728	U102	L536	G901-20	D212	D1466	U101	U121	B801
32.3	+++[b]	+++	+++	+++	+++	++	+++	+++	+++	+++	−	−	−	−	−
31.4	+++	+++	−	−	−	−	−	−	−	−	+++	+++	+++	+++	+++
31.5	+++	+++	−	−	−	−	−	−	−	−	−	−	−	−	−
30.2	−	+	+++	+++	+++	++	+++	+++	+++	+++	−	−	−	−	−

[a] S_2 = subunit of peplomer protein S.
[b] See legend (b) table I.

DISCUSSION

In an attempt to differentiate IBV variant strains, we prepared a panel of McAbs. McAbs to all structural proteins of IBV, except the S1 subunit, were obtained. The specificity of the McAbs could be easily determined in the immuno-electroblotting technique. Non-specific staining was not observed.

Evaluation of the cross-reactivity to IBV variant strains of the McAbs revealed that the McAbs specific for M and for N are directed to epitopes which are comon to almost all IBV strains. To the contrary, McAbs specific for S2 are directed to epitopes which are variably distributed among the variant strains. It is highly unlikely that the cross-reactivity of McAbs to M and to N should be explained because the variant strains are in fact identical, since the strains used in the test are claimed to belong to eleven distinct serotypes (Cowen, 1971; Hopkins, 1974; Cowen and Hitchner, 1975; Johnson and Marquardt, 1975; Darbyshire et al., 1979; Hofstad, 1981; Locher et al., 1983; Cook, 1984; Davelaar et al., 1984), and since the McAbs to S2 also differentiate a number of the strains. Because of the group-specificity, McAbs 25.1 to M and 26.2 to N are suitable for diagnostic purposes. Actually, we are using both McAbs for the detection of IBV-infected cells in an in vitro micro-neutralization test and in thin sections of organs of IBV-infected chickens.

The results suggest a difference in antigenic drift of the IBV structural proteins. No antigenic drift of M was observed thus far, as is apparent from the reactivity patterns of one cloned and 20 uncloned McAbs specific for M to the IBV variant strains (Table II and data not shown). The results suggest that N is also highly conserved. Two cloned and three uncloned McAbs to N reacted to all the variant strains with the exception of McAbs 26.2 and 26.3 which did not react to the SE-17 strain (Table II and data not shown). The number of McAbs with specificity for N, however, is to small to draw definitive conclusions. Furthermore, it should be stated that these conclusions are valid for one antigenic determinant of M and of N only, because formally it has not been proven, for instance by competition assays, that the 21 McAbs to M and 5 McAbs to N are directed to different epitopes. However, it is unlikely that all McAbs to M and to N have the same epitope specificity, in light of the heterogeneity of the antibody response.

Differences in optical densities of the reactions of McAbs directed to S2 were observed in the EIA, which could indicate differences in affinity of these McAbs for the strains. However, in the EIA the extent of the antibody-antigen reaction is dependent on antibody affinity, antibody concentration and density of the relevant antigen determinant (Steward and Lew, 1985). Particularly, the density of S determinants is difficult to control, because the amount of S varies between different isolates and even between different preparations of the same strain (Brown et al., 1984). The concentration of the S1 and S2 subunits could not be determined from the immunoblots, since the technique allows for qualitative interpretations only. Thus, the observed differences in optical densities can still be caused by differences in antigen concentration or in the affinity of the McAb for IBV variant strains. Therefore, only qualitative differences in the EIA are considered. Nevertheless, comparison of the reactivity patterns of different McAbs to the variant strains indicates that the affinity of some McAbs for different variant strains is variable. Considering these facts, the results permit the differentiation of variant strains. The grouping obtained by comparing the reactivity patterns of four McAbs to the Dutch variant strains is less discriminatory than the grouping according to results of the SN and HI tests. Up to now four serotypes have been proposed of which D207, D3128, D3896 and D212 represent the prototypes (Locher et al., 1983; Cook, 1984; Davelaar et al., 1984). Results obtained in the cross SN-test using reconvalescent sera showed close relationship between 0728, D274 and D207 and relationship to a varying extent between D212, D1466, U101 and B801 (Koch et al., submitted for publication). The McAbs did not make a distinction between the strains D207, D3128 and D3896. Possibly, these results indicate that the serotypes D207, D3128 and D3896 are more closely related to each other than to strains of the D212 serotype.

Some of the McAbs to S2 possessed in vitro neutralizing activity of virus infectivity. However, this activity was only observed with high concentrations of antibody present in ascites fluid. Furthermore, these McAbs neutralized other strains besides the homologous variant strain. Therefore we think that the observed neutralization is a consequence of the steric hindrance of virus infection by a high amount of antibody molecules bound to the virus and not by the binding of antibody to a region involved in neutralization. From this view our results support the observations of Mockett et al. (1984) and Cavanagh et al. (1984), which indicate the importance of the spike protein and in particular the S1 subunit in virus replication.

Recently, we obtained McAbs which showed high titres in the SN test. The cross-neutralization pattern of these McAbs permitted for the discrimination of more variant strains. Currently, we are determining the structural protein specificity of these McAbs.

ACKNOWLEGDEMENT
We thank Mrs. R. de Kok-Heuckeroth and J.C. Hoogeveen-Hilhorst for typing of the manuscript.

REFERENCES
Blore, P.J. and Skeeles, J.K. 1981. Use of a constant-virus diluting-serum microneutralization technique for the detection and quantification of

Infectious Bronchitis virus antibodies. Avian Dis. 25, 801-809.

Brodeur, B.R., Tsang, P. and Larose, Y. 1984. Parameters affecting ascites tumour formation in mice and monoclonal antibody production. J. Immunol. Meth. 71, 265-272.

Brown, T.D.K., Cavanagh, D. and Boursnell, M.E.G. 1984. Confirmation of the presence of avian Infectious Bronchitis virus (IBV) using cloned DNA complementary to the 3' terminus of the IBV genome. Avian Pathol. 13, 109-117.

Cavanagh, D. 1981. Structural polypeptides of coronavirus. J. gen. Virol. 53, 93-103.

Cavanagh, D. 1983a. Coronavirus IBV: further evidence that the surface projections are associated with two glycopolypeptides. J. gen. Virol. 64, 1787-1791.

Cavanagh, D. 1983b. Coronavirus IBV: structural characterization of the spike protein. J. gen. Virol. 64, 2577-2583.

Cavanagh, D., Darbyshire, J.H., Davis, P. and Peters, R.W. 1984. Induction of humoral neutralizing and haemagglutination-inhibiting antibody by spike protein of avian bronchitis virus. Avian Pathol. 13, 573-583.

Cook, J.K.A. 1984. The classification of new serotypes of Infectious Bronchitis virus isolated from the poultry flocks in Britain between 1981 and 1983. Avian Pathol. 13, 733-739.

Cowen, B.S., Hitchner, S.B. and Lucio, B. 1971. Avian Dis. 15, 518-526.

Cowen, B.S. and Hitchner, S.B. 1975. Serotyping of avian Infectious Bronchitis viruses by the virus-neutralization test. Avian Dis. 19, 583-595.

Darbyshire, J.H., Rowell, J.G., Cooke, J.K.A. and Peters, R.W. 1979. Taxonomic studies on strains of avian Infectious Bronchitis virus using neutralisation tests in tracheal organ cultures. Arch. Virol. 61, 227-238.

Davelaar, F.G., Kouwenhoven, B. and Burger, G.A. 1984. Occurrence and significance of Infectious Bronchitis virus variant strains in egg and broiler production in The Netherlands. Vet. Quarterly 6, 114-120.

Fazekas de St. Groth, S. and Scheidegger, D. 1980. Production of monoclonal antibodies: strategy and tactics. J. Immunol. Meth. 35, 1.

Hofstad, M.S. 1984. Avian Infectious Bronchitis. In: "Disease of Poultry" (Ed. M.S. Hofstad, B.W. Calnek, H.J. Barnes, W.M. Reid, and H.W. Yoder) (Iowa State Univ. Press, Ames, Iowa, USA). 8th edition. pp. 487-503.

Hofstad, M.S. 1981. Cross-immunity of chickens using seven isolates of avian Infectious Bronchitis virus. Avian Dis. 25, 650.

Hopkins, S.R. 1974. Serological comparison of strains of Infectious Bronchitis virus using plaque-purified isolants. Avian Dis. 18, 231-239.

Johnson, R.B. and Marquardt, W.W. 1975. The neutralizing characteristics of strains of Infectious Bronchitis virus as measured by the constant-virus variable-serum method in chicken tracheal cultures. Avian Dis. 19, 82-90.

Kearny, J.F., Radbuch, A., Liesegang, B. and Rajewsky, K.J. 1979. A new mouse myeloma cell line that has lost immunoglobulin expression but permits the construction of antibody-secreting hybrid cell lines. J. Immunol. 123, 1548-1550.

Köhler, G. and Milstein, C. 1975. Continuous cultures of fused cells secreting antibody of predefined specificity. Nature (London) 256, 495-497.

Locher, M., Lohr, J.E., Kosters, J., Kouwenhoven, B. and Davelaar, F.G. 1983. Vergleichende serologische Untersuchungen von süddeutschen Feldisolaten des Virus der Infektiosen Bronchitis der Hühner und den Holländischen Variantstammen D207, D3128 und D3896 in Trachealkulturen. Berl. Muench. Tierärtzl. Wschr. 96, 269-274.

Lomniczi, B. and Morser, J. 1981. Polypeptides of Infectious Bronchitis virus. I. Polypeptides of the virion. J. gen. Virol. 55, 155-164.

Lowry, O.H., Rosebrough, N.J., Farr, A.L. and Randell, R.J. 1951. Protein

138

measurements with the Folin phenol reagent. J. Biol. Chem. 193, 265-275.

Mockett, A.P.A., Cavanagh, D. and Brown, T.D.K. 1984. Monoclonal antibodies to the S1 spike and membrane proteins of avian Infectious Bronchitis virus coronavirus strain Massachusetts M41. J. gen. Virol. 65, 2281-2286.

Saunders, G.L. 1977. Development and evaluation of an enzyme-labeled antibody test for rapid detection of hog cholera antibodies. Am. J. Vet. Res. 38, 21-25.

Stern, D.F., Burgess, L. and Sefton, B.M. 1982. Structural analysis of virions proteins of the avian coronavirus Infectious Bronchitis virus. J. Virol. 42, 208-219.

Stern, D.F. and Sefton, B.M. 1982. Coronavirus proteins: Structure and function of the oligosaccharides of the avian Infectious Bronchitis virus. J. Virol. 44, 804-812.

Steward, M.W. and Lew, A.M. 1985. The importance of antibody affinity in the performance of immunoassays for antibody. J. Immunol. Meth. 78, 173-190.

Sturman, L.S. and Holmes, K.V. 1983. The molecular biology of coronaviruses. Adv. Virus Research 28, 35-112.

Van Zaane, D. and IJzerman, J. 1984. Monoclonal antibodies against bovine immunoglobulins and their use in isotype-specific ELISAs for rotavirus. J. Immunol. Meth. 72, 427-441.

EFFICIENCY OF OIL ADJUVANTED INFECTIOUS BRONCHITIS VACCINES

M. Guittet, V. Marius, J.P. Picault,
G. Bennejean, H. Lecoq, J. Lamande

Ministère de l'Agriculture, Direction de la Qualité, Services Vétérinaires
Laboratoire National de Pathologie Aviaire, B.P. 9, 22440 PLOUFRAGAN,
FRANCE

ABSTRACT

Four inactivated oil emulsion experimental and commercial infectious bronchitis vaccines were evaluated in non-vaccinated layers and in layers previously vaccinated with live vaccines, for their ability to increase the intensity and persistence of the immune response.

Experiments were performed on two specific pathogen free flocks which received only oil adjuvanted vaccines (OAV) and six conventional flocks previously vaccinated with live vaccines.

It is concluded that commercial OAV vaccines administered after live ones give better results in terms of both antibody responses and egg production. Revaccination of birds with H52 strain vaccine after a primary vaccination with H120 strain seems worthless if an oil adjuvanted vaccine is used for revaccination before lay.

INTRODUCTION

The ability of inactivated oil adjuvanted vaccines to prevent avian virus infections has been successfully demonstrated several years ago for Newcastle disease (ND), egg drop syndrome (EDS) and infectious bursal disease (IBD).

In the past, inactivated infectious bronchitis (I.B.) vaccines prepared with aluminium hydroxide adjuvant failed to protect birds under field conditions despite conclusive laboratory evidence of efficacy (Berry, 1965a, b, 1966; Box et al., 1966; Brion et al., 1969; Swarbrick et al., 1967). For this reason, studies have been carried out on the use of oil emulsions in the preparation of I.B. inactivated vaccines.

The development of these new I.B. vaccines led us to investigate their efficiency by both serological and challenge methods, and to evaluate their role in vaccination programmes for breeders and layers.

MATERIAL AND METHODS

Experimental birds and housing

Specific pathogen free (SPF) birds

Flock A : 52 twenty-three week old white Leghorn female breeders reared in isolators were housed in laying cages in separately ventilated rooms.

Flock B : 96 seventeen week old Warren pullets, previously reared in an isolated farm and serologically controlled for SPF status were transferred to laying cages in isolated rooms.

Conventional birds reared in field conditions until transferred or not to experimental units:

Flock C : 70 of 320 Warren pullets were transferred to experimental rooms at fourteen weeks old. The rest were moved at eighteen weeks old.

Flock D : 120 of 276 Warren and 36 Ross pullets from the same flock were transferred to experimental rooms at fourteen weeks old. The rest were moved at twenty weeks old.

Flock E : 125 fourteen week old Warren pullets were transferred to experimental rooms.

Flocks F, G, H : these three flocks were reared on the same farm throughout their life. F and H were laying flocks each containing 6 000 birds of different commercial breeds. G was a broiler breeder flock containing 3 500 birds of different breeds.

Vaccines and I.B. vaccination schedules

A number of different oil adjuvanted inactivated vaccines were studied. All were prepared with the Massachusetts strain and all except one were commercial products :

OAV_1 : monovalent experimental vaccine

OAV_2 : bivalent vaccine (I.B. + ND)

OAV_3 : monovalent vaccine

OAV_4 : trivalent vaccine (I.B. + N.D. + E.D.S.)

Inactivated I.B. vaccines were administered by intramuscular injection of 0.5 ml per bird.

Live vaccines were standard commercial bio-products : H 120, H 52, and MM strains administered by spray.

The different vaccination schedules are summarised in table 1 for flocks A and B, in table 2 for flocks C, D and E, in table 3 for flocks F, G and H.

Challenge

The I.B. virus challenge was the M 41 strain administered by different routes. The birds of flock C were challenged by the tracheal route with 10^3 EID50/0.2 ml per animal. The birds of flocks A and D were challenged both intra-tracheally with 10^3 EID50 per animal and by nebulisation with the

Atomist apparatus of 1.5 litres of virus suspension containing 10^8 EID50/ml. The birds of flocks B and E were challenged only by nebulisation as described above. The different ages at challenge are recorded in tables 1 and 2.

Serological monitoring

Before and at specified times after vaccination 20 birds per group were blood-sampled.

Serological tests

The haemagglutination inhibition (HI) test (Alexander and Chettle, 1977) was used to assess the antibody response to the I.B. component of the vaccines. Titres were expressed as the geometric mean of the reciprocal of the last dilution showing 100% inhibition. This test was run with 8 HA units of antigen (Mass. strain).

Egg production and egg quality

The egg production of each vaccinated group was recorded weekly before and after challenge by differentiating commercially usable and abnormal eggs. Statistical analysis were done by the X^2 method to study the percentage of lay and the percentage of abnormal eggs.

RESULTS

Serological responses

SPF birds flocks A, B (table 4)

The non vaccinated control birds showed no specific HI titres i.e. equal to 20. After one injection of oil I.B. vaccine, individual antibody titres reached 80 or 160 but the geometric means attained only 23 or 26 and decreased slowly thereafter. Following two injections the mean was a little higher i.e. 40.

Conventional birds in experimental conditions : flocks C, D, E, (Tables 5, 6, 7)

Comparisons of the different groups with equivalent vaccination schedules of these three flocks gave the following antibody titres during laying period.

- All the groups which received H 120 strain vaccines once or twice

TABLE 1 : Vaccination and challenge schedules : flocks A, B

Ages \ Flocks	A	B
22 weeks		OAV_4
23 "	OAV_2	
27 "	OAV_2	
28 "		←——— challenge ———→
33 "	←——— challenge ———→	

TABLE 3 : Vaccination schedules : flocks F, G, H

Ages \ Flocks	F	G	H
Hatching	H120	H120	H120
4 weeks	H120	H120	H120
12 "			H120
19 "	OAV_2		OAV_4
20 "		OAV_4	

TABLE 4 : Mean HI titres (range values) : Flocks A-B

Flocks	Groups	No of weeks after the last vaccination					
		-1	0	+3	+5	+6	+8
A	Vaccinated OAV2	23 (10-160)		40 (20-80)		30 (20-40)	
	Control un-vaccinated	10 (10)		10 (<5-20)		20 (20)	
B	Vaccinated OAV4		6 (5-10)	26 (10-80)	24 (20-40)		12 (10-20)
	Control un-vaccinated		6 (5-10)	5 (<5)	7 (5-10)		< 5 (<5)

TABLE 2 : Vaccination and challenge schedules : flocks C, D, E

Flocks		C				D				E			
Age	Groups	1	2	3	4	1	2	3	4	1	2	3	4
Hatching		H120	H120	H120	H120	H120	H120	H120	H120	H120	H120	H120	H120
4 weeks						H120	H120	H120	H120	H120	H120	H120	H120
14			H 52	H 52	H 52			H 52	H 52		H 52		H 52
18				MM	OAV 1		OAV 2		OAV 2			OAV 3	OAV 3
20													
28		← Challenge	Challenge	Challenge	Challenge								
29						← Challenge	Challenge	Challenge	Challenge				
31		← Challenge	Challenge	Challenge	Challenge					← Challenge	Challenge	Challenge	Challenge
40						← Challenge	Challenge	Challenge	Challenge				
42													

TABLE 5 : HI Titres : flock C

Groups	No of weeks after the last vaccination								
	0	3	4	6	7	8	12	17	20
H120	7 (5–40)		12 (10–20)	14 (10–40)	13 (10–40)	17 (10–40)	7 (5–20)	20 (10–40)	10 (5–20)
H120 H52	22 (10–320)		14 (5–80)			10 (5–20)	7 (5–20)	13 (10–40)	10 (5–40)
H120 H52 MM	22 (10–320)	54 (20–320)	22 (10–80)	14 (10–40)	10 (5–40)	9 (5–10)	15 (5–80)	27 (20–40)	19 (10–40)
H120 H52 OAV1	22 (10–320)	86 (20–640)	22 (10–80)	13 (10–20)	7 (5–10)	8 (5–10)	16 (5–40)	32 (10–80)	14 (5–40)

TABLE 6 : HI Titres : flock D

Groups	No of weeks after the last vaccination								
	0	9	12	15	17	19	22	26	29
H120x2	16 (10–40)	21 (10–40)	19 (10–40)	25 (10–40)	10 (5–20)	10 (5–20)	13 (10–20)		
H120x2 H52	20 (10–40)	28 (20–40)	16 (10–40)	12 (5–80)	9 (5–20)	13 (5–40)	14 (10–20)	9 (5–40)	10 (5–20)
H120x2 OAV2	16 (10–40)	37 (20–40)	40 (20–80)	98 (40–320)	28 (10–40)	61 (20–160)	32 (20–80)		
H120x2 H52 OAV2	20 (10–40)	37 (20–80)	43 (20–80)	23 (10–40)	28 (10–80)	46 (20–160)	44 (20–80)	30 (20–40)	44 (20–80)

TABLE 7 : HI Titres : flock E

Groups	No of weeks after the last vaccination				
	0	3	6	9	13
H120X2	6 (5–10)	6 (5–10)	10 (10)	7 (5–10)	5 (< 5–5)
H120x2 H52	49 (10–320)	53 (10–320)	70 (20–160)	25 (10–80)	13 (5–20)
H120x2 OAV3	6 (5–10)	171 (80–640)	211 (80–320)	130 (40–640)	46 (20–80)
H120x2 H52 OAV3	49 (10–320)	197 (80–640)	137 (40–640)	86 (20–320)	29 (10–40)

had low HI titres : the geometric mean did not exceed 25 and the highest
individual titre was 40.

- In groups revaccinated at 14 weeks with H52 strain vaccines the
geometric mean was not significantly higher than in the former groups
except for flock E in which individual titres rose up to 320.

- In flock C it can be observed that the 3rd vaccination at 20 weeks
old with MM strain did not modify the level of antibody compared to the
groups vaccinated with H 120 + H 52 strains.

- Difference was observed in groups revaccinated with different oil
emulsion vaccines. With the experimental vaccine (OAV$_1$) in flock C the
highest serological value observed was 86 three weeks after vaccination but
later no difference was observed compared with live vaccinated groups. The
vaccine OAV$_2$ in flock D generally gave higher antibody titres, on average
one more dilution than live vaccines. In flock E vaccinated OAV$_3$ groups
showed significantly higher HI titres.

Conventional birds in field conditions : flocks F, G, H (table 8)

These three flocks showed an I.B.-like clinical episode respectively
at 41, 17 and 30 weeks of age due to the coronavirus PL 84084. For flock F
the HI titres were not very high (i.e. 22, 38) despite the response seen at
forty-three weeks to infection with the variant virus.

In flock G the HI titres were higher than in flock F and remained at
the same level (66) during the life of birds.

In flock H the results were the highest of the three flocks ten weeks
after vaccination (90).

Egg production and egg quality results
SPF birds-flocks A, B (table 9)

After challenge highly significant differences in egg production and
quality were observed between the two groups : vaccinated and unvaccinated
controls. Nevertheless, there was a significant difference between
vaccinated challenge groups and unvaccinated non-challenge controls.

Conventional birds in experimental conditions : flocks C, D, E : (tables
10-11-12)

- Flock C : The comparison of both challenged or control birds showed
a very great difference for H120 vaccinated groups. For the other groups
significant differences were observed either at the 1st or 2nd challenge

TABLE 8 : HI titres : flocks F, G, H

Age (weeks) \ Flocks (vaccines)	F (OAV$_2$)	G (OAV$_4$)	H (OAV$_4$)
16		6 (< 5-20)	
19	7 (5-20)		7 (< 5-20)
22		65 (10-320)	
25		45 (20-80)	
27	41 (10-160)		
28			90 (80-320)
32	34 (10-80)	67 (40-160)	222 (80-640)
37	22 (10-80)		507 (160-1280)
38		66 (10-320)	
43	154 (20-320)		
44			249 (80-2560)
48		70 (20-640)	
51	38 (20-80)		
53			396 (160-2560)
56	22 (10-40)	40 (<5-160)	

TABLE 9 : Egg production and egg quality : flocks A, B

Flocks	Groups	Egg production % Challenge No	Egg production % Challenge Yes	Abnormal egg % Challenge No	Abnormal egg % Challenge Yes
A (5 weeks recording post challenge)	Control	71,72 a	40,97 b	0 d	12,38 e
	OAV$_2$ vaccinated		51 c		4,70 f
	Statistical analysis X 2	a c b (P < 0,01)		e f d (P < 0,01)	
B (10 weeks recording post challenge)	Control	90,05 a	60,72 b	0,2 d	10,61 e
	OAV$_4$ vaccinated		82,87 c		1,58 f
	Statistical analysis X 2	a c b (P < 0,001)		e f d (P < 0,001)	

TABLE 10 : Egg production % : flock C (8 weeks recording post challenges)

Groups ( )	1rst challenge		2nd challenge	
	No	Yes	No	Yes
H120 (a)	88,16	81,48	83,27	77,25
H120-H52 (b)	92,33	89,62	82,14	83;13
H120-H52-MM (c)	88,89	91,87	82,21	82,14
H120-H52-OAV$_1$ (d)	92,20	91,47	86,97	81,22
Comparison challenged /not challenged for each group	S (P<0,01) for a, b, c NS (P<0,5) for d		S (P<0,001) for a, d NS(P<0,5) for b, c	
Comparison unchallenged/groups	$\dfrac{\text{b d a c}}{\text{(P<0,01)}}$		$\dfrac{\text{d a b c}}{\text{(P<0,01)}}$	
Comparison of challenged groups	$\dfrac{\text{d c b a}}{\text{(P<0,01)}}$		$\dfrac{\text{b c d a}}{\text{(P<0,01)}}$	

TABLE 12 : Egg production and egg quality : flock E (4 weeks recording post challenge)

Groups ( )	Egg production %		Abnormal egg %	
	Challenge		Challenge	
	No	Yes	No	Yes
H120 x 2 (a)	92,14	77,15	O	19,18
H120 x 2 - H52 (b)	-	83,06	-	15,11
H120 x 2 - OAV$_3$ (c)	-	84,60	-	1,73
H120 x 2 -H52-OAV$_3$ (d)	-	87,55	-	2,66
Comparison not challenged/challenged for (a)	S (P<0,001)		S (P<0,001)	
Comparison of challenged groups	$\dfrac{\text{d c b a}}{\text{(P<0,05)}}$		$\dfrac{\text{a b d c}}{\text{(P<0,05)}}$	

S : Significantly different
NS : Not significantly different

TABLE 11 : Egg production and quality : flock D

Groups	Egg production % 1rst challenge (12 weeks recording)		Abnormal egg % (12 weeks recording)		Egg production % 2nd challenge (8 weeks recording)		Abnormal egg % (8 weeks recording)	
	No	Yes	No	Yes	No	Yes	No	Yes
H12O x 2 (a)	81,9	91,2	6,6	10,89		71,32		11,41
H12O x 2 - H52 (b)	90,1	86,7	4,1	12,13	81,88	79,68	4,67	8,02
H12O x 2 - OAV$_2$ (c)	91,4	89,1	9,8	12,57	-	77,48	-	10,49
H12O x 2 - H52-OAV$_2$ (d)	91,1	85,8	6	11,59	80,16	80,31	5,62	4,63
Comparison not challenged / challenged for each group	S (P<0,05) for b, c, d, (a not considered)		S (P<0,01) a, b, c, d		NS (P<0,05) for b, d		S (P<0,001) for b — NS (P<0,05) for d	
Comparison not challenged groups	c d b (P<0,05) (a not considered)		c a d b — P<0,001		b d (P<0,05)		d b (P<0,05)	
Comparison challenged groups	c b d (P<0,05) (a not considered)		c b d a (P<0,05)		d b c a (P<0,001)		a c b d (P<0,05)	

S : Significantly different
NS : Not significantly different

despite a slight decrease of egg production. Comparison of the challenge groups showed no difference between MM strain and OAV vaccines after the 1st challenge; after the 2nd challenge no difference was observed between the groups except for that receiving only H 120.

- Flock D : the lowest percentages of egg production in non-challenged groups was that of the H 120 vaccinated one and the highest in the challenged groups was the H120 vaccinated one. Because of our inability to explain this discrepancy, these 2 groups were discarded for statistical analysis.

At the 1st challenge highly significant differences were observed for egg production and egg quality between each challenged and non-challenged group. At the 2nd challenge no difference in egg production was recorded.

The best results in egg production after the 1st challenge were obtained with H120 plus OAV_2 vaccines. But after the 2nd challenge no differences were observed between groups revaccinated with either H52 or OAV_2 vaccines.

- Flock E : The H120 challenged and non-challenged groups were significantly different for egg production and egg quality. Comparison of the challenged groups showed that the OAV_4 vaccine provided the best results either associated or not with H52 strain vaccine. The production and quality data of flocks F, G, H which remained all their life under field conditions do not provide meaningful information. For flock G, which was exposed to the PL-84084 coronavirus before the laying period, production was as predicted, but for flocks F and H which were exposed after the peak of lay, drops in egg production were recorded. This was expected because this virus strain is antigenically different from Massachusetts.

DISCUSSION

According to Gough et al. (1977, 1981) mono, bi or trivalent inactivated IB vaccines stimulate similar immune responses.

The HI titres obtained in our experiments are lower than those of other authors (Gough et al, 1977; Box et al., 1980. 1981, 1985). This may be due to the fact that the HI test in France is performed with 8 HA units instead of 4 as in Great Britain. Moreover the values generally obtained with the HI test are lower than those obtained by beta-seroneutralisation (Marius et al., 1982; Renault et al., 1981).

In SPF birds, a poor primary response to inactivated emulsion vaccines was observed, confirming the results of Gough et al. (1977); the level of antibody was similar to that produced by live vaccines (Marius et al., 1982).

In conventional flocks C, D and E, to avoid the spread of H52 strain vaccine under field conditions, the groups not receiving this vaccine were transferred to isolated rooms just before vaccination of these flocks, so they were not infected. The HI titres obtained in groups receiving only live I.B. vaccines were similar to those observed previously (Marius et al., 1982). In the different vaccination schedules, the OAV I.B. vaccine was administered after live vaccines with a minimum of 4 or 6 weeks interval, taking into account the results of Box and Ellis (1985). The serological results of our experiments partially agree with those of Box and Ellis (1985) i.e. for the first point : the use of H52 strain vaccine before an oil emulsion vaccine does not appear to be necessary, but not for the second point : the best serological titres were observed when the OAV vaccine was administered 4 and not 6 weeks after the H52 one.

The different responses observed in antibody titres are probably due to the different vaccines. With the experimental OAV_1 vaccine a very short booster effect was produced and the level of antibody decreased rapidly. With OAV_2 vaccine a relatively low enhancing effect in HI antibody response was observed. Nevertheless the level persisted during the laying period under laboratory and field conditions (flocks D, F). OAV_3 and OAV_4 vaccines produced the highest rise in antibody titres. Furthermore these declined very slowly under laboratory conditions (flock E) and seemed to be persistent under field condition (flocks G, H).

The challenge experiments performed in the laboratory with virulent I.B. virus are helpful to appreciate the egg production in vaccinated groups.

In SPF birds the potency of OAV vaccine was indisputable although the protection was not entirely complete. Nevertheless OAV_4 induced better protection than OAV_2 vaccine.

In conventional birds, comparison of the egg production results obtained with the different vaccinated groups in which OAV vaccines were or were not used is difficult because several factors are involved :
– First : the severity of challenge is very important : a sharp drop of at least 30% in egg production has to be observed with the H120 alone vaccinated group in order to appreciate correctly the protection induced by the different revaccinations. To obtain this drop, nebulisation seems

to be the most appropriate route of challenge. This concerns flock E.

– Second : infection with even mild strains of field virus during the rearing period may possibly interfere with the immune response to vaccines.

– Third : the number of layers in experimental condition (24 to 36 maximum birds per group) is just on the limit to enable evaluation of the egg production.

– Fourth : For the flock D the different breeds of layers with different performances may explain the difficulties in interpreting the results.

Nevertheless, it can be concluded that after the 1st challenge the OAV vaccinated groups (whether they received H52 vaccine or not) showed the best results (except in flock D for which the challenge was not sufficient). After the 2nd challenge no difference was observed between revaccinated groups in which OAV vaccines are involved or not.

For egg quality our study was not as complete as these achieved by Protais et al. (1982), as only abnormal eggs were recorded. In SPF birds either OAV_2 or OAV_4 vaccines reduced the production of abnormal eggs after challenge. In conventional birds, if the flock D results are discarded, the best results were obtained with OAV_3 vaccine associated or not with H52 strain vaccine.

Although not as evident for egg production and egg quality as for HI responses, some differences between the ability of the different OAV vaccines to protect birds can be observed.

In conclusion, the efficacy of vaccination of breeders and layers before lay with I.B. oil adjuvanted vaccines seems demonstrated by the different experiments described in this study, despite the difficulties in estimating the protection with reference to the egg production data. With some of the OAV vaccines studied, better results were obtained after an initial vaccination with H120 strain. It must also be remembered that these experiments were concerned only with Mass types strain and not the variant I.B. strains.

REFERENCES

Alexander, D.J. and Chettle, N.J. 1977. Procedures for the haemagglutination and the haemagglutination inhibition tests for avian infectious bronchitis virus. Avian Pathology, 6, 9–17.

Berry, D.M. 1965a. Infectious Bronchitis and an Inactivated Infectious Bronchitis Vaccine. Spring Conference of the U.K. W.P.S.A. Branch, 277–283.

Berry, D.M. 1965b. Inactivated Infectious Bronchitis Vaccine. J. Comp.

Path., 75, 409–415.

Berry, D.M. 1966. Persistance des anticorps après vaccination avec le vaccin inactivé contre la Bronchite Infecteuse. Vet. Rec., 78, No 2, 81–83.

Box, P.G., Keeble, S.A., Berry, D.M. 1966. Expérience sur le terrain de l'emploi de vaccins inactivés pour la lutte contre la Maladie de New-castle et la Bronchite Infectieuse. Treizième Congrès International de volailles, Kiev, URSS.

Box, P.G., Beresford, A.V. and Roberts, B. 1980. Protection of laying hens against infectious bronchitis with inactivated emulsion vaccines. Vet. Rec., 106, 264–268.

Box, P.G., Roberts, B. and Beresford, A.V. 1981. Infectious bronchitis – preventing loss of egg production by emulsion vaccine at point of lay. International Symposium on Immunisation of Adult Birds with In-activated Oil Adjuvant Vaccines, Lyon, France. Development of Bio-logical Standards, 51, 97–103.

Box, P.G. and Ellis, K.P. 1985. Infectious bronchitis in laying hens : interference with response to emulsion vaccine by attenuated live vac-cine. Avian Pathology 14, 9–22.

Brion, A., Moraillon, A., Cakala, A. 1969. Valeur de la vaccination contre la Bronchitie Infectieuse aviaire par virus inactivé à la Beta-propiolactone. Recherches Vétérinaires, 2, 85–91.

Coria, M.F. 1972. Avian infectious bronchitis virus : serologic response of chickens to seven Beta -Propiolactone-inactivated strains. Avian diseases, 16, No 5, 1103–1108.

Gough, R.E., Allan, W.H. and Nedelciu, D. 1977. Immune response to mono-valent and bivalent Newcastle disease and infectious bronchitis in-activated vaccines. Avian Pathology, 6, 131–142.

Gough, R.E., Wyeth, P.J. and Bracewell, C.D. 1981. Immune responses of breeding chickens to trivalent oil emulsion vaccines responses to in-fectious bronchitis. Vet. Rec., 108, 99–101.

Guittet, M., Bennejean, G., Picault, J.P., Marius, V., 1984. Vaccins aviaires contre les affections respiratoires. Rec. de Méd. Vet., 160, No 11, 1085–1096.

McDougall, J.S. 1969. Avian infectious bronchitis : the protection afforded by an inactivated virus vaccine. Vet. Rec., 85, 378–381.

Marius, V., Guittet, M., Bennejean, G., 1982. Evaluation de l'immunité postvaccinale bronchite infectieuse chez des volailles élevées con-ventionnellement. Etude comparée de quatre techniques sérologiques. Av. Path., 11, 195–211.

Picault, J.P., Marius, V. 1984. La bronchite infectieuse aviaire. Rec. Med. Vet., 160, No 11, 939–950.

Protais, J., Marius, V., Guittet, M., Bougon, M. et Bennejean, G. 1982. Influence de la bronchite infectieuse sur la production et la qualité des oeufs. Bull. Inf. Stat. Exp. Avic., Ploufragan, 22, 71–86.

Swarbrick, O., Wyatt, A.R. and Leal, A.E. 1967. The use of inactivated in-fectious bronchitis vaccine in a large egg-production unit. Vet. Rec. 80, 273–277.

Renault, L., Deshayes, A., Alamagny, A., Marius, V., Guittet, M., Bennejean, G. 1981. Diagnostic et contrôle de la vaccination de la bronchite in-fectieuse aviaire. Bull. Soc. Vet. Prat., France, 65, 1–11.

EVALUATION OF VACCINATION EXPERIMENTS IN BROILER BREEDERS AND LAYERS WITH LIVE VIRUS AND FORMALIN INACTIVATED OIL EMULSION INFECTIOUS BRONCHITIS VACCINES

E. F. Kaleta, C. Cegla

Institut fur Geflugelkrankheiten
Justus-Liebig-Universitat
Frankfurter Str. 87
D-6300 Giessen
Federal Republic of Germany

ABSTRACT

Data of a serological survey indicate that approximately 2/3 of 131 random samples (equivalent to 2,405 sera) contain HI antibodies to Massachusetts and variant IB viruses. Vaccination experiments prove that live plus inactivated Massachusetts-type vaccination provides reliable and long lasting protection against homologous field virus challenge. Vaccination with a single dose of inactivated oil emulsion variant virus results in poor sero-conversion and little if any protection against field challenge with virulent variant viruses. The priming of chickens with attenuated live variant viruses during the growing period is strongly recommended.

INTRODUCTION

Avian infectious bronchitis virus (IBV) has caused health and egg production problems for years in laying and meat type chickens due to affections of the (i) respiratory tract, (ii) urogenital tract, mainly in kidney and uterus and (iii) intestinal tract (Davelaar et al., 1981, 1983; Cook, 1984; Protais et al., 1982). Clinically similar disease entities can be induced by more than ten serotypes/variants of IBV (Johnson, 1976; Cowen, 1975; Davelaar et al., 1983; Lutticken, 1983; Hopkins, 1974).

To control the various forms of the disease two main approaches seem to be feasible. Choice number one could be the selection and use of vaccine viruses which have a very broad antigenicity and provide protection against homologous and heterologous challenge with nearly all serotypes. Choice number two would be the development of multivalent vaccines which contain vaccine viruses of all major IBV serotypes/variants. Presently the latter approach seems to be more realistic.

We describe in this paper results of a serological survey which includes the most wide spread Massachusetts (M-41) serotype and two more recently detected serotypes/variants (ref. strain Nos. D-274 and D-1466). The vaccination experiments under field conditions were performed with presently available Massachusetts-type live virus vaccines and an inactivated oil emulsion vaccine which contains M-41 and two variant viruses.

MATERIALS AND METHODS

Specified details of chicken flocks, vaccines and methods used will be described elsewhere (Cegla, 1985, manuscript in preparation).

Serological survey

Random samples ranging on an average of 18 sera per submission originated from laying flocks and broiler stock. All sera were heat inactivated prior to testing.

Vaccines

Commercially available live virus vaccines containing either H-120 or H-52 Massachusetts-type virus were used either as spray at day-old or as eye-drop or drinking-water-method according to the recommendation of the manufacturers. The oil emulsion vaccine (Intervet, NL) contained M-41, D-274 and D-1466 viruses.

HI test

The hemagglutinating antigens from M-41, D-274 and D-1466 viruses were produced according to generally accepted procedures (Alexander et al., 1976, 1977, 1983; Lutticken, 1983).

RESULTS

Serological survey

A total of 131 random samples, equivalent to 2,405 sera were tested. Only 18 random samples did not contain detectable amounts of HI antibodies to M-41, D-274 and D-1466. The majority of random samples contained HI antibodies against M-41 and variant viruses. Only rarely mono-infections with variant viruses could be detected (Table 1).

Vaccination experiments

The main results of the vaccination trial are summarized in Table 2. The use of M-41 virus either as live or in addition to inactivated virus did entirely prevent clinical disease caused by this serotype in the 20

TABLE 1   Number of submitted random samples (Jan. 1983 – Feb. 1985) tested for HI antibodies against antigens (M-41, D-274 and D-1466) tabulated according to geographical origin of samples (total of 131 random samples).

a = 2000 north to 8000 south part of West-Germany

b = Mean of IBV-HI titre of random sample < 4 log 2

c = Mean of IBV-HI titre of random sample $\geqq$ 4 log 2

M-41	D-274	D-1466	n	%	No. of tested random samples from postal zip code area (a)						
					2000	3000	4000	5000	6000	7000	8000
- (b)	-	-	18	13,7	1		9		7	1	
+ (c)	-	-	28	21,5	2	2	11	1	9		3
+	+	-	47	35,9	3	7	24		13		
+	+	+	29	22,1	1	3	13	3	9		
-	+	+	1	0,8				1			
-	-	+	0	0,0							
+	-	+	4	3,0	2				2		
-	+	-	4	3,0			1		3		

TABLE 2   IBV vaccinations, serology and IB associated clinical symptoms in 19 chicken flocks.

- = IBV-HI titre (log 2) ≤ 4   / = not done, not tested, not observed
+ = IBV-HI titre (log 2) > 4   x = formalin inactivated oil emulsion vac.
# = IBV-HI titre (log 2) > 7   xx = spray vaccination at 1 day of life

Flock	IBV-Vaccination at weeks			IBV-Antibody Status at			post 3.IB-vac. to			IB Problems at weeks of life		Possible Field Infection with
	H-120	H-52	OE^x	M-41	D-274	D-1466	M-41	D-274	D-1466	egg-drop/shell sympt.	respir. sympt.	
A	4	11	22	-	-	-	+	-	-	29	29	D-274
B	4	11	22	+	-	-	+	-	-	29	29	D-274
C	4	11	22	+	-	-	+	-	-	50	50	D-274
D	3	10	20	-	-	-	+	-	-	27	27	D-274 and/or D-1466
E	3	10	20	-	-	-	+	-	-	27	27	"
F	3	10	20	+	-	-	+	-	-	27	27	"
G	3	10	20	-	-	-	+	-	-	27	27	"
H	3	3/	/	/	/	/	/	/	/	/	9	D-274
I	3	10	20	-	-	-	+	-	-	/	/	/
2	1d^{xx}	7	16	#	+	+	+	+	+	/	/	/
5	1d	10	22	#	#	#	+	+	+	/	9	D-274
6	1d	9	21	+	-	-	+	-	-	/	/	/
8	1d	8	15	-	-	-	+	-	-	42	42	D-274
10	1d	8	15	+	+	+	+	+	-	/	/	/
1	1d	7/15/	/	+	+	+	+	+	+	/	/	/
3	1d	7/15/	/	+	+	+	+	+	+	/	/	/
4	1d	9/15/	/	/	/	/	+	+	+	59	59	D-1466
7	1d	8/21/	/	+	-	-	+	-	-	/	/	/
9	1d	9/15/	/	+	+	-	+	+	-	/	/	/

flocks examined. In addition, M-41-live virus priming and subsequent booster with inactivated homologous virus did induce high and uniform HI antibodies. The mode of application, e.g. spray, eye-drop, drinking-water or
injection is obviously not of paramount importance for protection in comparison to live virus priming.

The oil emulsion vaccine contained also the variant viruses D-274 and
D-1466. If field infection with these viruses occured during the growing
period, antibodies were boostered by the inactivated vaccine and persisted
throughout the production period. No clinical disease was observed in these
cases.

On the contrary, first and only application of inactivated variant virus antigen did not provide persisting HI antibodies and long-lasting resistance to homologous field virus challenge.

The clinical data indicate that variant virus field infection may result either in egg-production disorders or in a combination of this with
respiratory symptoms (Table 2).

DISCUSSION

The data of the field survey emphasise once more the wide-spread occurrence of the variant viruses in layer and meat type chickens. Most if not
all of the M-41 positive random samples originated from flocks vaccinated
with H-120 and/or H-52 viruses.

The vaccination experiments prove that live plus inactivated vaccines
provide adequate protection against challenge with homologous viruses. One
vaccination with inactivated variant viruses is of minor and short-lived
value. In these cases also live virus priming is a prerequisite for reliable and long-lasting immunity. The introduction of attenuated live variant viruses into the chicken population does not pose a health risk because
- as the serological survey indicates - virulent variant viruses are widely
distributed in intensively maintained chicken flocks.

REFERENCES

Alexander, D.J., Bracewell, C.D. and Gough, R.E. 1976. Preliminary evaluation of the haemagglutination and haemagglutination inhibition tests
for avian infectious bronchitis virus. Avian Pathol., 5, 125-134.
Alexander, D.J. and Chettle, N.J. 1977. Procedures for the haemagglutination and the haemagglutination inhibition tests for avian infectious
bronchitis virus. Avian Pathol., 6, 9-17.
Alexander, D.J., Allan, W.H., Biggs, P.M., Bracewell, C.D., Darbyshire,
J.H., Dawson, P.S., Harris, A.H., Jordan, F.T.W., Macpherson, I.,

McFerran, J.B., Randall, C.J., Stuart, J.C., Swarbrick, O. and Wilding, G.P. 1983. A standard technique for haemagglutination inhibition tests for antibodies to avian infectious bronchitis virus. Veterinary Record, 113, 64.

Cook, J.K.A. 1984. The classification of new serotypes of infectious bronchitis virus isolated from poultry flocks in Britain between 1981 and 1983. Avian Pathol., 13, 733-741.

Cowen, B.S. and Hitchner, S.B. 1975. Serotyping of avian infectious bronchitis viruses by the virus-neutraluzation test. Avian Dis., 19, 583-595.

Davelaar, F.G., Kouwenhoven, B. and Burger, A.G. 1983. Experience with vaccination against infectious bronchitis broilers and significance of and vaccination against IB-variant viruses in breeders and layers in the Netherlands. La Clinica Veterinaria, 106, 8-11.

Davelaar, F.G., Kouwenhoven, B. and Burger, A.G. 1984. Occurrence and significance of infectious bronchitis virus variant strains in egg and broiler production in the Netherlands. Veterinary Quarterly, 6, 114-120.

Hopkins, S.R. 1974. Serological comparisons of strains of infectious bronchitis virus using plaque-purified isolants. Avian Dis., 18, 231-239.

Johnson, R.B. and Marquardt, W.W. 1976. Strains of infectious bronchitis virus on the Delmarva peninsula and in Arkansas. Avian Dis., 20, 382-386.

Lütticken, D. 1983. Significance of variant infectious bronchitis serotypes in the Netherlands. West. Poultry Conf. California, USA.

Lütticken, D. and Cornelissen, D.R.W. 1984. Use of the haemagglutination inhibition test for antibodies to avian IB-variant strains. 17th World's Poultry Congr. Helsinki, Finnland. Scientific Papers, 4. Hygiene and Path., 525-527.

Protais, J. Marius, V., Guittet, M., Bougon, M. and Bennejean, G. 1982. Effect of infectious bronchitis on egg production and quality. Bulletin d'Information Station Expérimentale d'Aviculture de Ploufragen, 22, 71-72; 75-86.

PRELIMINARY RESULTS WITH A COMBINED INACTIVATED NEWCASTLE DISEASE
AND INFECTIOUS BRONCHITIS (VARIANT STRAIN) VACCINE IN LAYING HENS

V. Papparella
Department of Pathology, Prophylaxis and Inspection of Meats,
Avian Pathology Section,
Veterinary Faculty, Via F. Delpino, 1-80137 Napoli, Italy

ABSTRACT

This paper reports a booster effect obtained under field conditions
by using a combined inactivated Newcastle disease and infectious bronchitis
vaccine containing the classic M and two Dutch variant (D274 and D1466)
infectious bronchitis virus serotypes. An additional vaccination at 16
weeks of age with this vaccine gave a superior level of immunity to that
obtained using only live vaccines.

In Italy, infectious bronchitis (IB), because of the continuous
emergence of new serotypes, continues to cause egg production problems,
particularly in areas with intensive production. The purpose of this
paper is to report preliminary results of a booster effect obtained under
field conditions by using a combined Newcastle disease and IB vaccine.
This vaccine is an oil adjuvanted inactivated commercial product (Intervet.
Nobivac IB3 + ND), containing the classic Massachussetts and two Dutch
variant (D 274 and D 1466) IB virus serotypes. Evidence of the presence
of the variant serotypes in Italy has been obtained by Marchi and Zanella
(1984).

A total of 3,000 birds was used. Day old chicks were spray vaccinated
with IB (H120) vaccine. At 2 weeks of age, they were vaccinated via the
drinking water with the La Sota strain of Newcastle disease virus. At 6
weeks they received D 274 and at 10 weeks D 1466, both by the nasal route.
Live IB vaccines were supplied by Intervet. At 16 weeks of age, 2,500
birds were vaccinated with the combined inactivated Newcastle disease and
IB vaccine (0.5 ml subcutaneously in the neck). Five hundred birds were
used as controls to verify any booster effect. After a further 3 weeks,
10% of each group of birds were bled and pooled samples were used to
determine antibody titres to Newcastle disease and IB viruses.

The results (Table 1) show that in areas where the variant IB strains
are present, a booster vaccination at 16 weeks of age with the combined
inactivated vaccine gave a superior level of immunity to that obtained
using only live vaccines. Further work to determine the persistence
of these antibodies is in progress.

TABLE 1   ANTIBODY TITRES THREE WEEKS AFTER VACCINATION WITH
           COMBINED INACTIVATED VACCINE

	Antibody titre ($_2$log) against			
	Mass IB[a]	D274 IB[b]	D1466[b]	Newcastle disease virus[b]
Birds boosted with combined inactivated vaccine	6.5	6.2	7.4	7.8
Control birds (live vaccines only)	4.1	4.6	5.8	4.6

(a) Neutralisation test in SPF eggs using constant serum: varying
     virus method.

(b) Haemagglutination inhibition test.

REFERENCES

Marchi, R. and Zanella, A. 1984. Bronchite infettiva aviare: isolamento
    di un sierotipo apparentemente nuovo del virus e sua diffusione.
    La Clinica Veterinaria, 107, 121-125.

AN ENTEROTROPIC AVIAN INFECTIOUS BRONCHITIS VIRUS

R.C. Jones [1], M.El Houadfi[2], Jane K.A. Cook [3], and A. Ambali. [1]

[1] Sub-Department of Avian Medicine, University of Liverpool,
Leahurst, Neston, Wirral, L64 7TE, England.
[2] Institute Agromonique et Veterinaire
Hassan II, Rabat, Morocco.
[3] Houghton Poultry Research Station, Houghton,
Huntingdon, Cambs, PE17 2DA, England.

ABSTRACT

Of six isolates of infectious bronchitis (IB) virus isolated from commercial poultry flocks in Morocco, five (designated D,E,F, H and M) were related serologically to the Massachusetts serotype, while a sixth, (designated G) was found to be different from any previously reported serotype of IB virus. Neutralising antibodies to this virus have been detected in the sera of commercial chicken flocks from a number of regions in Britain. While isolate G, in common with the other 5 isolates, caused respiratory disease typical of IB in 3-week old SPF chicks, it showed a particular predilection for the alimentary tract, and at various times up to 28 days could be isolated from all regions between oesophagus and bursa of Fabricus. Greatest persistence occurred in the anterior regions (oesophagus, proventriculus and duodenum).

INTRODUCTION

As part of an investigation into the nature of viruses involved in respiratory disease in chicken flocks in Morocco, six isolates of IB virus have been characterised (El Houadfi and Jones, 1985). This paper draws particular attention to one of the isolates, designated G which appears to be serologically unusual and enterotropic.

MATERIALS AND METHODS

All isolations were made from chicken flocks in the Rabat-Temara region of Morocco. Five of the agents (D,F,G,H and M) were isolated from respiratory disease in broilers, none of which were vaccinated against IB, and the sixth (E) was from a 25-week old commercial laying flock which was given H52 vaccine in the drinking water at 15 weeks. In 5 cases isolations were made after 1-3 passages of respiratory material in 9 day-old fertile eggs, but isolate G required 5 passages. Isolates were characterised as IB virus based on morphology under the electron microscope, responses to treatment with chloroform, pH 2.9, heating at 56 °C, and demonstration of IB virus group antigen by ELISA. Cross-neutralisation tests were done in tracheal organ cultures to compare the isolates with the major British, American, Australian, Dutch and other European serotypes of IB virus (see Cook 1984 for viruses).

The pathogenicity of the six viruses was tested by intranasal infection of 3-week old SPF chicks, and the virus persistence in trachea, kidney and rectal contents determined by virus isolation in SPF eggs. A second experiment investigated the persistence of virus G in different regions of the alimentary tract over a 28 day period.

RESULTS

Biophysical properties:

All six isolates were characterised as IB viruses by having typical coronavirus morphology, were sensitive to chloroform, resistant to low pH, had variable heat resistance, and possessed the IB virus group antigen.

Serological relationships:

Five of the isolates were broadly related by cross-neutralisation to Massachusetts (M41) serotype and H120 and H52 vaccine viruses. Isolate G was unrelated to the other 5 Moroccan viruses and showed no serological relationship in either direction with any of the reference laboratory or field strains tested.

Incidence of antibodies to virus "G" in Britain:

Neutralising antibodies to isolate "G" were found in 8/30 breeder flocks and 5/16 commercial laying flocks. Serological evidence of infection was widespread, being found as far afield as Scotland (North), Hampshire (South), Norfolk (East) and Wales (West). Antibodies were detected in sera collected in 1978. Of 21 flocks with antibodies to any of the Dutch Serotypes D207, D212, D3128, or D3896, 11 were positive for isolate G also while 10 were negative. None had antibodies to G only.

Pathogenicity experiments:

All 6 isolates induced mild respiratory disease in 3-week old SPF chicks, and microscopic changes in tracheas were typical of IB.

Virus persistence in tissues:

Results of all 6 isolates are shown in Table 1, where the striking feature is the long persistence of isolate G in the lower intestine, although it was not detected in trachea or kidney beyond day 9.

TABLE 1. Persistence of 6 Moroccan IB viruses in the trachea, kidney or lower intestine of SPF chicks infected intranasally at 3-weeks of age.

Virus	Trachea	Kidney	Lower Intestine
D	9a	-	-
E	14	14	
F	14	-	9
G	9	9	28
H	14	-	-
M	14	-	-

a: last day virus isolated between days 7-28

Table 2 shows that isolate G could be detected at all levels of the alimentary tract at various times during the 28 day experiment. Ileum, caecal tonsil and bursa were positive as early as day 3 but the anterior regions (oesophagus, proventriculus and duodenum) showed greater persistence of virus in the later stages.

TABLE 2. Isolation of Moroccan IB virus isolate G from various regions of the alimentary tract, and from trachea and kidney of SPF 3-week old chicks at intervals after infection.

Tissues Examined	Days after infection					
	3	7	10	14	21	28
Oesophagus	-	-	+	+	+	-
Proventriculus	-	+	+	+	+	-
Duodenum	-	+	-	+	+	+
Jejunum	-	-	+	-	-	-
Ileum	+	+	+	-	-	-
Caecal Tonsils	+	+	+	-	-	-
Bursa of Fabricius	+	+	-	+	-	-
Cloacal swabs	-	+	+	+	+	+
Trachea	+	+	-	-	-	-
Kidney	-	+	+	+	-	-

+: Virus isolated from pooled tissue from 3 birds.
-: no virus isolated.

DISCUSSION

While all 6 Moroccan IB virus isolates induced respiratory disease in SPF chickens typical of IB, virus neutralisation tests separated the five related to the Massachusetts serotype (isolates D,E,F,H and M) from isolate G which is serologically unique, and has a particular predilection for the alimentary tract.

Virus G was initially the most difficult of the agents to isolate, requiring 5 passages in eggs before it caused typical embryo effects. This may perhaps explain why it has not yet been isolated from flocks in Britain despite serological evidence of its presence. The latter fact propably means that viruses related to G are present in other parts of Western Europe. Indeed isolate G might in time prove to be related to one of the IB variants reported elsewhere.

With regard to the enterotropism of virus G, reference has been made by others to persistence of IB viruses in the alimentary tract (Cook, 1968; Alexander and Gough, 1977), although results have usually been based on examination of tissues at the posterior end of the gut or cloacal swabbing. Other evidence supporting the potential susceptibility of different regions of the gut to IB virus has been presented by the in vitro organ culture studies of Darbyshire and others (1976 & 1978). However, no detailed study of the pathogenesis for the alimentary tract of IB viruses such as G has been done, and current experiments are underway to determine which cells of the gut are infected, and whether infection in very young chicks will cause digestive malfunctioning.

At present the significance of isolate G is unknown but a preliminary vaccine trial in young chicks has indicated that H120 vaccination appear to be ineffective (El Houadfi and others, to be published).

REFERENCES

Alexander, D.J. and Gough, R.E. (1977). Isolation of infectious bronchitis virus from experimentally infected chickens. Research in Veterinary Science 23: 344-347.

Cook, J.K.A. (1968). Duration of experimental infectious bronchitis in chickens. Research in Veterinary Science 9: 506-514.

Cook, J.K.A. (1984). The classification of new serotypes of infectious bronchitis virus isolated from poultry flocks in Britain between 1981 and 1983. Avian Pathology 13: 733-741.

Darbyshire, J.H., Cook, J.K.A. and Peters, R.W. (1976). Organ culture studies on the efficiency of infection of chicken tissues with avian infectious bronchitis virus. British Journal of Experimental Pathology 57: 443-454.

Darbyshire, J.H., Cook, J.K.A. and Peters, R.W. (1978). Growth comparisons of avian infectious bronchitis virus strains in organ cultures of chicken tissue. Archives of Virology 56: 317-325.

El Houadfi, M. and Jones, R.C. (1985). Isolation of avian infectious bronchitis viruses in Morocco including an enterotropic variant. Veterinary Record 116: 445.

RUNTING IN BROILERS

B. Kouwenhoven, M.H. Vertommen and E. Goren.

Poultry Health Institute
P.O. Box 43, 3940 AA Doorn
The Netherlands

ABSTRACT

The main symptoms and pathological changes of the runting and stunting (malabsorption) syndrome as they are observed in many countries are described. Criteria used to define successful experimental infections are formulated.

Results of experimental work are presented from which it appeared that runting is an infectious condition in which the intestine is the target organ. Birds developed all clinical and pathological aspects of the syndrome only if they were infected during the first days of life. The main spread of the infectious agent(s) is horizontally and it occurs very rapidly. Although vertical transmission is suggested by circumstantial evidence, this has not been proved.

While a viral aetiology was suspected, attempts to reproduce the disease with reoviruses and coronaviruses isolated from field cases were unsuccessful. The original theory of a viral aetiology was questioned when it appeared that the pathogenicity of a diluted homogenate could be sedimented by low speed centrifugation. Moreover in a series of 3 bird passages of a bacteria-free filtrate of the homogenate, the pathogenicity decreased rather than increased.

The syndrome could be reproduced by inoculation of a combination of isolated aerobic and anaerobic bacteria and a bacteria-free filtrate, but not with each of these inocula separately. These results indicate involvement of both virus(es) and bacteria(e) in the aetiology.

General features of the disease

Runting and stunting, a disease of mainly broilers but sometimes also of broiler breeders, was described for the first time approximately 8 years ago in The Netherlands. Since then identical or similar syndromes have been observed in broilers in other European and non European countries (Belgium, England, N. Ireland, Italy, Denmark, German Federal Republic, Spain, The Near East, Australia, Mexico, South America, USA). There are also reports of the syndrome in turkeys. These observations indicate a worldwide distribution of the disease. While it seems to come and go "in waves", in many areas runting is the most important cause of economic loss in broiler production.

Clinically the disease combines the non-specific characteristics of several different diseases such as impaired growth and bad feathering. However the presence of many, sometimes up to 20 per cent, birds that seem

not to grow at all, is characteristic of the runting syndrome. This can
be observed from as early as 5 days of age. At 6 weeks birds can still have
the appearance of a chick just a few days old and they weigh less than
100 g. A varying fraction of such birds shows feathering abnormalities.
The replacement of down, especially at the head, is retarded, leading to
"yellow heads". Feather growth is poor and wing feathers may point to
different directions, causing an appearance called "helicopter chicks".

The excretion of yellow-orange, wet to mucoid droppings in which much
maldigested feed is present, has also not been observed in other diseases.
The yellow droppings are observed only when birds are fed a diet containing
yellow corn or carotenoid pigments in another form. Then also another
criterion, ie the presence of birds with pale shanks, can be observed.

At necropsy, pale swollen small intestines with thin liquid maldigested contents and sometimes gas accumulation are found up to an age of
2 weeks. Microscopically by day 3 and 7 necrotic and cystic changes are
observed in the Lieberkühn glands of the small intestine. Thereafter up
to about 3 weeks of age, the main changes are multilayering of the intestinal epithelium and the presence of great numbers of goblet cells, indicating a metaplasia of the epithelial cells to mucus producing cells.
Proventriculitis (Kouwenhoven et al., 1978) is definitely not a part of
the syndrome; it should be regarded as a completely separate cause of
growth retardation.

From 2 - 3 weeks of age a large proportion of birds develop changes
of rachitis and/or osteoporosis of the rapidly growing bones such as tibia
and femur. Widened epiphyseal growth lines can be seen macroscopically on
longitudinal sections of the proximal parts of these bones. More rarely,
there is a hyaline enlargement of the tuberculae and capitulae costarum.

While pancreatic fibrosis is thought to be a part of the disease in
England and Australia, this has not been observed in other countries.

Both experimentally and in field cases the disease goes together with
long lasting serum concentrations of carotenes and fat soluble vitamins A,
D and E. (Encephalomalacia, due to low vitamin E concentration, can also
be an aspect of the syndrome). The alkaline phosphatase (ALP) activity in
the serum is increased up to about 4 weeks pi and it could be demonstrated
that this was most likely of intestinal origin.

In experimental studies described below a successful infection was
determined by a combination of growth impairment up to 3 weeks after

infection of one-day-old chicks, excretion of yellow-orange mucoid to wet droppings from approximately day 4 up to 3 weeks pi, an increased plasma ALP activity and decreased carotenoid concentration up to 3-4 weeks pi and macroscopically widened epiphyseal growth plates of the proximal tibia 3-4 weeks pi.

The infectious nature of the syndrome was demonstrated by experimental reproduction of all its characteristics by oral administration of intestinal homogenates to one-day-old broiler chicks kept in isolators. The syndrome could again be reproduced with intestinal homogenates made from these birds 2 weeks after infection and so on. These observations, together with the clinical symptoms (diarrhoea, decreased carotene plasma concentrations) make it most likely that the digestive tract is the primary target for the infectious agent.

An extensive series of experiments has been carried out in order to study the infectiosity, the epidemiology and spread of the infection and the etiology.

To some of the questions we can give quite a detailed answer. However, with respect to the etiology the definite answer cannot be given (at least not by us today), but we can give some indications.

Epidemiology and spread of the disease

So far the disease has been observed mainly in broilers. There have been some cases in broiler breeders. This means that it is a disease of the heavy fast growing breeds. The disease is even connected with the growth rate. Symptoms after experimental infection were less serious in broilers kept on layer feed than in birds that were forced to grow fast on broiler feed. This shows that the syndrome is a typical luxury disease of the fast growing chick.

Although there is circumstantial evidence pointing to vertical transmission of the infection, there is no experimental proof of it.

Age related resistance

An important observation concerning the epidemiology was an age related resistance; the younger the birds, the more sensitive they are to the infection. So when significant pathological changes are present then the infection has taken place at a very young age. This is illustrated in Table 1. Although birds inoculated at 7 days of age developed general

TABLE 1   Influence of age at infection on disease parameters

Infected at	Body weight	Day 29 ALP	Bone changes
Day 1	680	1100	Yes
Day 7	790	438	No
Day 14	978	n.d.	No
Uninfected	977	n.d.	No
Day 1	472		Yes
Day 3	688		No
Uninfected	716		No

disease symptoms, especially diarrhoea (from day 21 (= day 14 pi) until day 29 even more than those infected at one-day old), they contracted no bone abnormalities. It is remarkable that in these birds the ALP activity was low at day 29 in contrast to that in the birds infected at one-day old. So obviously bone disorders develop only when pathological changes take place (in the intestine) during the first days of life. In this connection it is remarkable that mineralization in the normal broilers used in these experiments, does not take place before the 7th or 8th day of life. In-oculation at 14 days of life did not result in any clinical symptom nor in bone changes. In another experiment depicted in Table 1 there was a great difference even between inoculation at an age of one day or at three days. The latter birds obviously are already much less sensitive to the disease than the day-olds (just hatched).

Spread of the disease

The disease spreads easily and apparently very rapidly. This is shown in Table 2. When birds were placed in contact and 50% or 25% were infected, the contact birds acquired the disease 100%. They suffered at least as much from the syndrome as the infected birds. They also developed bone changes at least as much and to the same extent as the infected birds. Since we have seen that after infection at 3 days of age no bone abnormalities developed and that also weight losses were much smaller than after infection at one day of age, it can be concluded only that infection spreads very rapidly from one bird to another, most likely within one day.

TABLE 2   Spread of the infection

	Isolator	Body weight	Day 22 ALP	Bone changes
A.	60 birds inoculated	379	1747	+
B.	30 birds inoculated	377		+
	30 birds not inoculated	349	2747	+
C.	60 birds not inoculated	627	499	−
D.	10 birds inoculated			
	30 birds not inoculated	210	2100	+
E.	40 birds not inoculated	425	500	−

Etiology

Reoviruses

The disease was reproduced to a certain degree with bacterium-free 450 and 220 nm filtrates as shown in Table 3.

TABLE 3   Effect of filtration and treatment with reovirus hyper-immune serum

	Body weight	Day 19 Carotene	ALP	Osteoporosis
Homogenate	366	0.43	1641	+
450 nm	436	0.57	1826	+
220 nm	436	0.46	1153	+
Homogenate + broth	424	0.46	1340	+
Homogenate + anti REO	444	0.14	958	+

Since then the attention was directed to a viral etiology.

From all field cases we investigated, a reovirus was isolated and from experimentally infected birds reovirus was isolated from the intestines (or faeces) even 5 weeks after oral inoculation with the crude homogenate.

However, with none out of 8 different reoviruses that were isolated from 8 different infectious homogenates, was it possible to reproduce the syndrome. These isolates were from 7 Dutch field cases and one Italian.

On the other hand reoviruses were more or less pathogenic after oral inoculation. They caused a more or less serious diarrhoea during 1-2

weeks. However, this diarrhoea was not of the yellowish mucoid type.
Birds excreted watery sometimes mucoid faeces which had a grey black colour
like normal faeces; sometimes it was a little yellow.

Table 4 gives the parameters of a typical reovirus infection as compared with infection with a crude homogenate. It is clear that reovirus
caused a temporary growth retardation. However, even after 2 weeks the
difference with the uninfected birds was over. Equally the increased ALP
activity and the decreased carotenoid concentration was over by 3 weeks.
This is in contrast to the birds inoculated with the infected homogenate.
Here ALP and carotenes were still high/low at 4 weeks of age. So these
parameters were changed for 2 weeks longer than in the reovirus infected
birds.

We also infected with intestinal homogenate from reovirus infected
birds, without success (bird passage).

TABLE 4   Comparison of reovirus and crude homogenate

Age (days)	Reovirus			Infected homogenate			Uninfected		
	Body wt.	ALP	Car.	Body wt.	ALP	Car.	Body wt.	ALP	Car.
3 days	58	1357	2.1	51	1232	1.5	61	864	2.1
1 week	97	3473	0.35	59	1486	0.37	122	1238	0.71
2 weeks	247	1731	0.43	129	2534	0.19	318	1122	0.57
3 weeks	499	684	0.65	214	1988	0.16	501	650	0.50
4 weeks	761	615	0.45	501	1009	0.14	785	397	0.35
	No Osteoporosis			Osteoporosis			No Osteoporosis		

In another important experiment (Table 3) the crude inoculum was
treated for some hours with an anti reovirus hyperimmune serum and an equal
volume as a control with broth. From the antiserum-treated inoculum reovirus could not be isolated (not even after 23 CKC passages); from the
broth treated inoculum it was readily isolated. Equally from the intestines
from inoculated birds reovirus was isolated/not isolated at 7 and 14 days
after infection. However, with both inocula the disease was reproduced to
the same extent, although not completely. So obviously the absence of reovirus in the inoculum did not mean the absence of infectiosity. However,
there are also results of an experiment that revealed, in contrast with the
results just mentioned, some role for reovirus (Table 5).

TABLE 5   Influence of reovirus infection at day-old

Inoculation	Body weight	Bone changes
Homogenate day 1	472	Yes
Homogenate day 3	688	No
Reo day 1 + homogenate day 3	540	Yes
Reo day 1	592	No
Not inoculated	716	No

Birds were inoculated at 3 days of age and they developed practically no symptoms (weight loss, bone abnormalities) as compared with control birds inoculated at day 1. But when birds had been infected at day-old with reovirus, they developed the complete syndrome after inoculation at day 3, although the growth retardation in the day-old infected group was still significantly greater than in the reo 1 + crude 3 inoculated group. The weight loss in this group was mainly due to reovirus which alone produced a significant weight loss but no bone abnormalities. This role of reovirus acting as a trigger or a preinfection could not clearly be established in another experiment. So we concluded that reovirus as such cannot cause the disease but that an early infection with reovirus under some unknown conditions may facilitate infection with the true agent.

Viruses other than reoviruses

We isolated some adenoviruses. They were of no pathological significance.

After treatment of our standard crude inoculum with anti reovirus serum we isolated both from the inoculum and from the intestine of infected birds a virus which proved to be a coronavirus. This isolate, designated B29C5, on experimental infection caused diarrhoea and weight loss comparable with that caused by the crude inoculum. But this diarrhoea was, although mucoid and wet, not yellow enough. ALP activity was increased until day 21 but 4 days later it was normal and so was the carotene concentration. However in 4 out of 29 infected birds we observed ribknob swelling. In a further experiment (Table 6), the virus used had been adapted to growth in the allantoic sac. It had undergone 15 embryo passages (5 yolk sac and 10 all. sac) and had a titre of $10^{6.2}$ EID50. This amount was inoculated in experimental birds. These birds developed a long lasting diarrhoea and weight loss, longer than in the control infected birds. But in these birds the diarrhoea was mucoid and yellow which was not the case in the birds inoculated with the isolate.

Birds did not develop bone abnormalities which were present in the controls. It can be seen also that neither ALP values nor carotene concentrations showed significant changes in this group, again in contrast with the infected controls. Also birds developed antibody against B29C5 after infection with this isolate but not with the crude inoculum from which it was isolated.

TABLE 6   Comparison of B29C5 coronavirus and crude homogenate

| | Day 22 | | | | Day 50 |
	Body w.	ALP	Carot.	Bone abnorm.	Antibodies to B29C5
Uninfected	743	low	high	-	No
Crude homogenate	590	high	low	+	No
B29C5 coronavirus	585	low	high	-	Yes

In the next series of experiments it was attempted to remove the coronavirus from the intestinal homogenate by incubation with an antiserum. In these experiments an incubation step for 30 minutes followed by centrifugation at 3000 g was also involved and the supernatants were used as inoculum. Experimental infections showed that the pathogenicity of such supernatants had decreased considerably. However the pathogenicity of homogenates after similar treatment with saline (inoculated control groups) had decreased to the same extent. A possible explanation for these results was sought in the effect of the centrifugation, keeping in mind that the centrifugal force and time applied was too low to sediment viruses.

A most important finding was obtained in further experiments, as presented in Table 7. Centrifugation was again for 30 minutes at 3000 g and 4°C. Birds in group 3 were slightly ill only at day 4 and 5 pi and they excreted some yellow faeces. In contrast birds in the inoculated groups 4, 5 and 6 were seriously ill from day 2 through 12 or 14 pi during which time they excreted typically yellow mucoid dropping. The clinical picture in these groups was the same and much more serious than that in group 3,

173

TABLE 7 Effect of centrifugation of crude homogenate

Group	1	2	3	4	5	6
Treatment	Infected control	Uninf. control	Supernatant of homogenate 1 vol. + saline 4 vols. after centrif.	Sediment of homogenate 1 vol. + saline 4 vols. after centrif.	Supernatant as in 3 + sediment as in 4, re-combined	Homogenate 1 vol. + saline 4 vols. Not centrif.
Body weight	345[+]	708	523	360	415	386
ALP	1763	706	2404	3482	2106	2692
Carotene	0.063	0.345	0.274	0.160	0.161	0.105
Bone changes	13/13*	0/16	10/16 (slight)	14/15	14/14	14/14

[+]All parameters measured at 22 days pi

*Number of birds with changes in the proximal tibia/number examined

174

but slightly milder than that in group 1.

From this experiment it was concluded that the pathogenicity of an inoculum consisting of a crude intestinal homogenate diluted 1:5 in saline could be sedimented easily for the greatest part by centrifugation for only 30 minutes at a relatively low centrifugal force of 3000 g and that after recombination of the more pathogenic sediment and the less pathogenic supernatant, pathogenicity was recovered.

These results pointed strongly to involvement of bacteria in the etiology or of a virus that could be sedimented as easily as bacteria, eg attached to easily sedimented particles. Regarding the latter, one thinks of eg rotaviruses. Sera taken from broilers 7 weeks after experimental inoculation with a pathogenic homogenate, had no antibodies against rotavirus.

In order to clearly define the significance of any virus present in the supernatant in the etiology, the experiments presented in Tables 8, 9 and 10 were carried out. The principle was simple: if any virus were the causative agent, it would be present in a 450 nm filtrate, hence this filtrate would be pathogenic on its own, or at least it would be pathogenic in a subsequent second or third bird passage. This pathogenicity would increase rather than decrease during these bird passages. The filtrate

TABLE 8   Effect of filtration of crude homogenate

Group Treatment	1 None	2 450 nm filtrate (1st bird passage)	3 Crude homogenate
Body weight	319[+]	255	143
ALP	760	3933	3176
Carotene	0.618	0.302	0.123
Bone changes*	1	2	4

[+]All parameters measured at day 14 pi.
*Maximum score can be 4.

used (Table 8) was made by centrifuging the homogenate for 30 minutes at 3000 g, passing the supernatant through a 450 nm filter, centrifuging again for 10 minutes at 3000 g (the small amount of sediment produced proved bacteriologically sterile) and passing this supernatant again through a 450 nm filter. From this filtrate a reovirus was easily isolated.

It appears from Table 8 that the control birds inoculated with crude homogenate displayed all parameters of full pathogenicity. The filtrate, although pathogenic, caused retardation, lowered carotene concentrations and bone deformations that were intermediate between those of the inoculated and uninoculated control birds. Five birds showed a great growth inhibition, 24 were moderately inhibited. The ALP activities in this group were higher than in the inoculated control birds.

Intestines were collected from 8 birds of group 1 and 3 and inoculated in groups 1 and 3 of the next experiment (Table 9). From 4 birds of group 2 that showed the greatest growth inhibition, intestines were collected separately from those of 8 other birds that had shown the intermediate grade of growth inhibition. From these intestines also homogenates were made and inoculated in groups 2.a and 2.b (Table 9).

It appears clearly that the filtrate had lost pathogenicity by the second bird passage. This observation reduced the possibility of a virus as the only causative agent considerably. If it were a virus, pathogenicity should have increased during the first bird passage.

In the experiments presented in Table 10 the intestinal homogenates made from birds of group 2.b (Table 9) were inoculated in birds of group 2, representing a third bird passage. The birds in group 1 were inoculated with intestinal homogenates made from the birds of group 1, Table 9, representing a second bird passage of intestinal homogenate from not inoculated birds. Carotene concentrations are not presented. It appears that in a third bird passage of filtrate made from the original homogenate, pathogenicity again has not increased. From this series of experiments it was concluded that a virus could be excluded as the primary and only causative agent of the runting and stunting (mabsorption) syndrome.

The involvement of bacteria or of bacteria and viruses was then investigated. Both aerobic and anaerobic bacteria were isolated from intestines 3 days after infection with the crude homogenate. It was attempted to reproduce the disease with these bacteria or with a combination of a bacteria-free filtrate as before, plus a mixture of these bacteria. The filtrate was supposed to contain any virus (reovirus and coronavirus were present, possibly others also). The bacterial part of the inoculum was composed of hundreds of different colonies. The bacteria were not identified. No virus could be isolated from this bacterial inoculum.

The main results are presented in Table 11 from which appears that the filtrate caused a limited growth inhibition as before and also a limited

TABLE 9   Effect of passage in birds on pathogenicity of filtered crude homogenate

Group Treatment		Homogenate uninf. control birds group 1 (Table 8) 1st bird pass.	Homogenate smallest bird group 2 (Table 8) 2nd bird pass.	Homogenate intermed. birds group 2 (Table 8) 2nd bird pass.	Homogenate control birds group 3 (Table 8) 2nd bird pass.	Inoculated control	Not inoculated control
Body weight	Inoculated(15)*	397+	332	300	212	124	361 (25)
	Contact (10)	411	347	313	217	154	
ALP	Inoculated	983	3036	2547	3768	1187	542
Carotene	Inoculated	0.409	0.314	0.355	0.140	0.134	0.573
ALP	Contact	846	2121	2412	4179	1558	
Carotene	Contact	0.384	0.334	0.345	0.119	0.116	
Bone changes	Inoculated	0	0.4	1.1	2.4	1.9	0
	Contact	0	0.3	1.25	2.3	2.7	

*( ) number of birds

+All parameters measured at day 17 pi

TABLE 10 Effect of passage in birds on pathogenicity of filtered crude homogenate

Group Treatment		1 Homogenate group 1, Table 9 2nd bird pass. not inoculated	2 Homogenate group 2.b Table 9 3rd bird pass. filtr.	3 None	4 Inoculated Controls
Body weight	Inoculated (15)* Contact (10)	334+ 334	306 267	407	166 142
ALP	Inoculated Contact	1345 1243	1408 986	794	1674 1224
Bone changes	Inoculated Contact	0.3 0.6	0.1 0.9	0.27	1.2 1.7

* ( ) number of birds

+ At day 16 pi

TABLE 11   Investigation of involvement of bacteria in etiology of runting.

Group		1	2	3	4	5
Treatment		Filtrate	Filtrate + bacteria	Bacteria	Crude homogenate	None
Body weight	Inoculated	398[+](19)[*]	299(19)	411(20)	294(19)	478(21)
	Contact	408 (5)	297(5)	355(5)	314 (5)	544(5)
ALP	Inoculated	1469	1411	740	1085	722
	Contact	1688	1207	1161	1873	617
Carotene	Inoculated	0.563	0.352	0.660	0.234	0.993
	Contact	0.709	0.346	0.630	0.254	0.908
Bone changes		0.42	0.84	0.76	1.44	0.46

[*] ( ) number of birds.
[+] Measured at day 20 pi.

decreased carotene concentration. The ALP activity was like that in the inoculated control group. Equally the birds inoculated with the bacteria showed about the same slight changes.

In contrast the bacteria and filtrate together caused a growth inhibition and ALP values that were the same as in the inoculated control group. The carotene concentrations were also considerably lower than in the birds inoculated with bacteria or filtrate only and not much higher than in the inoculated controls. Birds in group 2 excreted yellow coloured mucoid faeces like the birds in group 4 until about 14 days pi. Bone changes in group 2 were less than in group 4.

It can be concluded that in this experiment the syndrome was almost completely reproduced by inoculation of a bacteria-free filtrate of an infectious homogenate plus various bacteria isolated from intestines of birds at day 3 pi. These results confirmed our theory based on experiments described above that the etiological agent could not be a 450 nm filtrate agent only, but that a bacterial component was also involved.

REFERENCE

Kouwenhoven, B., Davelaar, F.G. and van Walsum, J. 1978. Infectious proventriculitis causing runting in broilers. Avian Pathol. 7, 183-187.

RUNTING SYNDROME IN BROILER CHICKENS. EXPERIMENTAL REPRODUCTION STUDIES

G. Meulemans, M. Decaesstecker, G. Charlier

National Institute for Veterinary Research
99, Groeselenberg
1180 Brussels, Belgium

ABSTRACT

SPF white leghorn and commercial broiler chickens were orally infected at 1 day old with a field material containing an entero-like virus together with a reovirus; a reovirus, an entero-like virus and a parvovirus alone. Abnormal faeces and reduction in weight gains were observed after infection with the field material or the entero-like virus. No clinical signs nor growth retardation were observed in day-old SPF and commercial broiler chickens orally infected with reo or parvoviruses. SPF white leghorn chickens were found as susceptible as commercial broiler chickens for the study of weight gain depression after oral inoculation at one day of age.

INTRODUCTION

Several viruses including reovirus, rotavirus, parvovirus and enterolike viruses have been detected in the faeces of broilers affected by the runting/malabsorption syndrome. (Van der Heide et al., 1981; Page et al., 1982; Hieronymus et al., 1983; Mc Ferran et al., 1983; Mc Nulty et al., 1984; Kisary et al., 1984; Kisary, 1985).

The aetiological role of these different viruses is still nowadays questionable.

From previous experiments it seems unlikely that rotaviruses act as aetiological agents in the runting/malabsorption syndrome (Meulemans et al., 1985).

This paper describes the clinical observations recorded after oral inoculation of day-old SPF white leghorn and commercial broiler chickens with a field material containing an entero-like virus together with a reovirus; a reovirus, an entero-like virus and a chicken parvovirus alone.

MATERIALS AND METHODS

A. Field material

1. Stock preparation

Intestinal contents from 10 days-old broilers showing runting
were collected and made into a 25 % suspension in TNE pH 8.7
(Tris 0.01M, NaCl 0,1M, EDTA 0.001M) and administrated orally
to 1 day old SPF chickens (Valo, Lohmann) held in isolators.
Seven days later, these birds were killed and their intestinal
contents collected, pooled and made into a 25% suspension in
TNE pH 8.7. The suspension was freezed and thawed and clarified
by centrifugation at 10.000g for 30 minutes at 4ºC. The supernatant was removed and stored at -20ºC. This constituted our
field material stock.

2. Electron microscopic examination

Using the method C of Mc Nulty et al. (1979), we could show
in this field material preparation the presence of numerous
small round unenvelopped entero-like virus particles (mean
diameter 32 nm) together with a reovirus (fig. 1).

B. Reovirus

1. Stock preparation

The reovirus used came from chicken embryo liver cells inoculated
with the field material stock.
After three passages in these cells, the supernatant was collected and stored at -20ºC. This constituted our reovirus stock.

2. Reovirus identification

The reovirus was identified by electron microscopy (fig. 1)
and by direct immunofluorescence using a fluorescein conjugate
antiserum to the EK 1133 strain of Van der Heide (Meulemans
et al., 1980).

C. Entero-like virus

1. Stocks preparations

The field material preparation was pelleted through a 45% sucrose
cushion at 100.000g for 90 minutes at 4ºC. The pellet was resus-

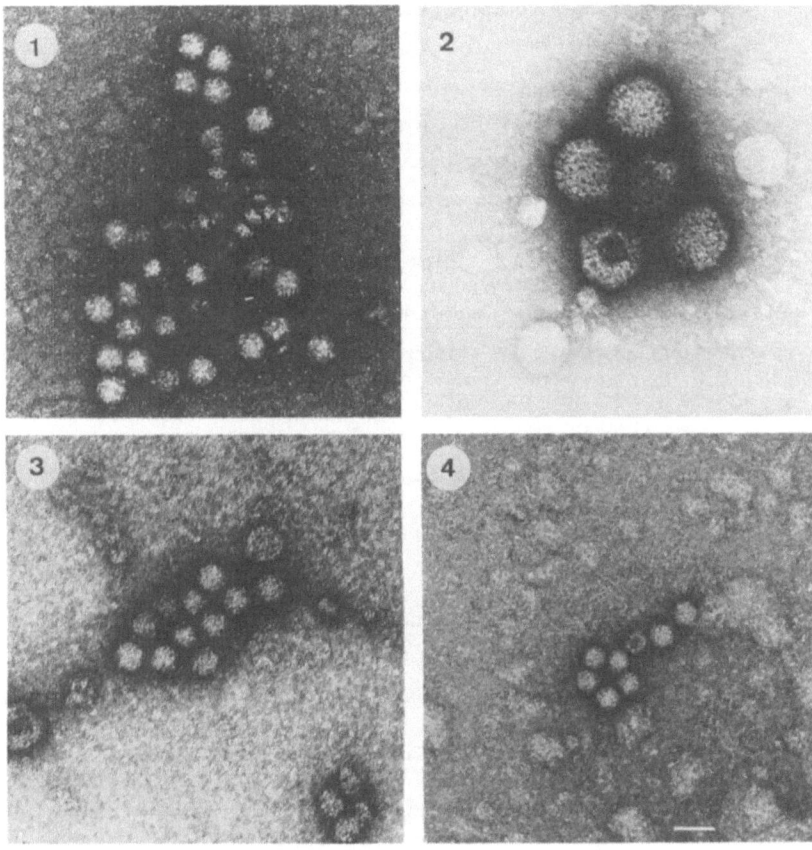

Fig. 1 : Viruses detected in stocks preparations by direct electron microscopy Bar represents 50 nm

1. Entero-like virus particles from field material

2. Reovirus isolated in cell culture

3. Entero-like virus particles from entero-like virus preparation

4. Parvovirus particles from parvovirus preparation

pended in TNE in 1/60 of the starting volume and passed through a 50 nm Millipore filter. Day-old SPF chickens were inoculated orally with 100 μl of the filtrate and killed 7 days later; their intestinal contents were collected and treated as described for the field material. Using this first preparation, three serial passages were successively made by oral inoculation in day-old SPF chickens. The supernatants from the centrifugated intestinal suspensions obtained after each passage were stored at -20°C and designated entero-like virus stock preparations number 1, 2 and 3.

2. Electron microscopic examination

Numerous entero-like virus particles were seen in all stock preparations (fig. 1).

3. Control of absence of other viruses in the stocks

The different entero-like virus preparations were inoculated on chicken embryo liver and kidney cells.

No cytopathic effect was observed after 3 passages in these cells what demonstrated the absence of the reovirus initially present in the field material.

The entero-like virus preparation number 2 was pelleted through a 45 % sucrose cushion at 100.000g for 90 minutes at 4°C. The pellet was resuspended in TNE in 1/90 of the starting volume and submitted to isopycnic density gradient centrifugation in CsCl d 1.36 at 80.000g for 65 hours at 4°C. After fractionation of the gradient in 60 μl aliquots, all fractions having a density between 1.31 and 1.43 were examined by electron microscopy after negative staining. Entero-like virus particles were observed at a density of 1.35 - 1.37, no other virus was found.

D. Parvovirus

1. Stock preparation

The chicken parvovirus used was the ABU strain received from J. Kisary (Kisary et al., 1984).

The virus was first purified after multiplication in day-old

SPF chickens infected orally. At eight days of age, the chickens were killed and their intestines were collected, pooled and made into a 25% suspension in TNE. The suspension was freezed and thawed 3 times and clarified by centrifugation at 10.000g during 30 minutes at 4°C. The supernatant was removed and pelleted through a 45% sucrose cushion at 100.000g during 90 minutes at 4°C. The pellet was resuspended in TNE in 1/100 of the starting volume, treated with CH_3Cl (V/V) and centrifugated at 1200g during 10 minutes. The aqueous phase was removed and submitted to isopycnic density gradient centrifugation in CsCl, d 1.41 at 130.000g for 72 hours at 4°C. After fractionation of the gradient in 60 μl aliquots, all fractions having a density between d 1.36 and 1.44 were examined by electron microscopy after negative staining. Virus particles with the typical morphology of parvoviridae were observed at d 1.42 (full particles) and d 1.36 (empty particles). A stock preparation of parvovirus was made by inoculation of day-old SPF chickens with the d 1.42 particles. The chickens were killed 8 days later and their intestinal contents collected, pooled and treated as described for the field material.

2. Electron microscopic examination

This preparation was shown to contain numerous parvovirus particles (diameter 19 - 22 nm) (fig. 1).

3. Parvovirus serology

Antibodies against parvovirus were searched using the Elisa test performed following the already described procedure (Meulemans and Halen, 1982). CsCl purified parvovirus was dialyzed against TNE buffer, treated with KSCN 2M (V/V) (Inouye et al., 1984) during 15 minutes and diluted 1/10 in carbonate/bicarbonate buffer pH 9.6. Before testing, the sera were absorbed with avian SPF faeces (10 % w/v) and diluted 1/100. A positive reference serum (OD = 540) obtained by immunization of SPF birds with the ABU strain and a negative serum (OD = 80) were included in all tests.

E.   Experimental infections

One day-old white leghorn SPF chickens (Valo Lohmann) and commercial broiler chickens were used as experimental subjects. The chickens were inoculated orally with 100 μl of the different inocula. Control groups were uninoculated chickens of the same origin. All birds were weighed at 1 day and observed during 7 to 21 days. Birds were weighed and necropsied at different times intervals as reported in tables 1 and 2. All birds were housed on wire floor in isolators fitted with absolute filters at air entry and exit points. They were fed using a commercial broiler starting meal containing 22% proteins. The growth retardation was calculated using the following formula :

$$\text{growth retardation \%} = \frac{\text{weight gain controls - weight gain infected}}{\text{weight gain controls}}$$

RESULTS

A.   Field material

SPF and broiler chickens inoculated orally at 1 day of age started to pass abnormal faeces within 2 days after inoculation and this lasted for a period of about 8 days. Some chickens had cloacal pasting at 5-7 days of age. Inoculated chickens were more uneven and smaller than controls (Tables 1 and 2). Growth retardation was more important during the first week after inoculation than later on.

Paleness of the small intestine was observed at necropsy performed at 7 days. No feather changes as helicopter chickens, bone abnormalities or increased mortality were observed.

At 7 days of age, entero-like virus and reovirus particles were detected in the faeces of inoculated birds.

B.   Reovirus

No clinical signs nor growth retardation (table 1) were observed in day-old SPF chickens infected orally. The reovirus was reisolated at 7 days of age from the faeces of the inoculated birds.

C.   Entero-like virus

SPF and broiler chickens inoculated orally at 1 day of age showed the clinical signs observed and reported for the field material.

TABLE 1   Weights and growth retardation of SPF chickens after oral inoculation at 1 day old

Experimental groups	Weight in grams			% growth retardation	
	1 day	7 days	14 days	1 to 7 days	7 to 14 days
Field material (10 ♀, 10 ♂)	39,34ᵃ ± 2,73ᵇ (35,8 - 43,7)	58,29 ± 6,12 (50 - 65)	109,43 ± 10,06 (95,3 - 129,5)	50,62	16,67
Controls (13 ♀, 8 ♂)	40,29 ± 3,23 (34,4 - 47,5)	78,48 ± 6,53 (73 - 95)	139,85 ± 15,57 (102,5 - 173,6)		
Reovirus (8 ♀, 10 ♂)	40,36 ± 4,02 (35,2 - 50,6)	81,20 ± 6,75 (70,5 - 93,0)	-	0	-
Controls (11 ♀, 5 ♂)	39,41 ± 3,63 (35,1 - 48,6)	75,66 ± 8,11 (59,9 - 87,0)			
Entero stock II (7 ♀, 10 ♂)	34,71 ± 2,49 (30,2 - 38,1)	54,59 ± 7,20 (36,7 - 70,8)	-	42,37	-
Controls (11 ♀, 6 ♂)	33,77 ± 2,23 (28,8 - 37,8)	68,27 ± 6,17 (55,4 - 83,5)			
Entero stock III (8 ♀, 12 ♂)	43,08 ± 4,13 (31,5 - 47,2)	68,73 ± 9,23 (52,0 - 78,6)	-	31,08	-
Controls (8 ♀, 11 ♂)	43,18 ± 3,34 (37,3 - 49,7)	80,40 ± 5,62 (70,8 - 87,3)			
Parvovirus (6 ♀, 9 ♂)	41,90 ± 2,46 (37,4 - 44,6)	79,52 ± 4,77 (69,9 - 87,6)	-	0	-
Controls (12 ♀, 2 ♂)	42,22 ± 3,56 (35,9 - 48,4)	76,21 ± 6,95 (64,8 - 92,2)			

a Mean weight ± standard deviation
b Range of weights

TABLE 2 Weights and growth retardation of broiler chickens after oral inoculation at 1 day old

Experimental groups	Weight in grams				% growth retardation		
	1 day	7 days	14 days	21 days	1 to 7 days	7 to 14 days	14 to 21 days
Field material (100 ♂)	33,92[a] ± 3,82 (29,3[b] – 41,3)	115,83 ± 15,23 (89,7 – 147,7)	294,72 ± 46,81 (193 – 369)	575,3 ± 79,63 (343 – 739)	24,88	9,76	4,25
Entero stock II (100 ♂)	33,83 ± 4,83 (30,1 – 40,6)	117,90 ± 15,78 (88,7 – 164,1)	305,96 ± 38,38 (192 – 380)	584,34 ± 63,97 (460 – 790)	22,91	5,13	5
Controls (100 ♂)	34,28 ± 2,26 (29,9 – 41,8)	143,32 ± 11,43 (115,9 – 161,8)	341,56 ± 29,98 (237 – 392)	634,60 ± 78,18 (527 – 755)			
Parvovirus (75 ♂)	36,96 ± 3,46 (28,5 – 44,4)	129,07 ± 14,47 (86 – 156)	–	–		–	
Controls (75 ♂)	36,91 ± 3,22 (31,6 – 45,7)	124,90 ± 14,56 (95 – 162)	–	–	0		
Parvovirus from CsCl gradient (75 ♂)	34,25 ± 2,76 (27,41 – 39,15)	162,25[c] ± 16,13 (128 – 192)	392,67[d] ± 24,70 (355 – 440)	660,33 ± 46,69 (545 – 675)	0	0	0
Controls (75 ♂)	35,4 ± 3,28 (30 – 43,9)	163,47[c] ± 19,47 (102 – 191)	385,00[d] ± 25,14 (340 – 425)	647,00 ± 77,34 (440 – 770)	0	0	0

a Mean weight ± standard deviation
b Range of weights
c Weight at 8 days
d Weight at 15 days

186

Growth retardation observed after inoculation with the entero-like virus alone was comparable to this observed after inoculation of the field material which contained entero and reovirus (tables 1 and 2). Entero-like virus particles were observed in the faeces, 7 days after infection.

D.   Parvovirus

No clinical signs nor growth retardation were observed in day-old SPF and broiler chickens infected orally (tables 1 and 2). In each experiment, parvovirus was detected in the faeces of the infected birds, 7 days after infection.

Serological testing of broiler chickens used in experimental infection trials showed the absence of parvovirus antibodies in the serum of the day-old chickens; O.D. values of tested sera were always less than those of negative control sera.

DISCUSSION

In our experiments, it has been possible to reproduce at least in part, the runting syndrome by oral inoculation of field material containing an entero-like virus associated with a reovirus or with an entero-like virus alone into day-old SPF or broiler chickens. These results confirm and extend the findings of Mc Nulty et al. (1984) who postulated that destruction by entero-like virus of villous intestinal cells in the small intestine results in a malabsorption type diarrhoea which leads to the decrease in weight gains.

In contrast, no growth retardation nor clinical signs were observed after oral infection of day-old SPF and broiler chickens with reo or parvoviruses.

The growth retardation observed after inoculation of field material or entero-like virus alone varied between 22 and 50 %. As runting results from malabsorption, modifications in the composition of the food used in experimental work could account for these variations between different trials.

The growth retardation that has been observed during the second and third weeks of age in the inoculated chickens was less obvious than during the first week of age suggesting the effect is temporary. For this reason, we limited the observation period in some of our experiments to the first week after infection.

No bone changes nor feather aberrations were produced after infection with field material or entero-like virus but these are rare in the natural disease in Belgium.

SPF white leghorn chickens were found as susceptible as broiler chickens for the study of weight gain depression after oral inoculation at one day of age. Therefore, we would recommend their use to avoid the possibility of interference with maternal antibodies or the contamination of day-old chickens by vertical transmission of enterovirus as described by Spackman et al. (1984).

ACKNOWLEDGEMENTS

The skilfull technical assistance of Mrs M.C. Carlier and M. Raeymaekers is gratefully acknowledged.

REFERENCES

Mc Ferran, J.B., Mc Nulty, M.S., Mc Cracken, R.M., Greene, J. 1983. Enteritis and associated problems. In : The International Union of Immunological Societies Proceeding n° 66 : Disease Prevention and Control in Poultry Production, pp 129-138. Edite by Hungerford, T.G., Sydney : University of Sydney.

Hieronymus, D.R.K., Villegas, P., Kleven, S.H. 1983. Identification and serological differentiation of several reovirus strains isolated from chickens with suspected malabsorption syndrome. Avian Dis., 27, 246-254.

Inouye, S., Matsumo, S., Yamaguchi, H. 1984. Efficient coating of the solid phase with rotavirus antigens for enzyme-linked immunosorbent assay of immunoglobulin A antibody in feces. Jnl. of Clin. Microbiol., 19, 259-263.

Kisary, J., Nagy, B., Bitay, Z. 1984. Presence of parvoviruses in the intestine of chickens showing stunting syndrome. Avian Path., 13, 339-343.

Kisary, J. 1985. Experimental infection of chicken embryos and day-old chickens with parvovirus of chicken origin. Avian Path., 14, 1-7.

Meulemans, G., Froyman, R., Halen, P. 1980. Epidémiologie des maladies virales des poulets de chair. 1. Les affections à Réovirus. Ann. Méd. Vét., 124, 513-519.

Meulemans, G., Halen, P. 1982. Enzyme-linked immunosorbent assay (Elisa) for detecting infectious laryngotracheitis viral antibodies in chicken serum. Avian Path., 11, 361-368.

Meulemans, G., Peeters, J.E., Halen, P. 1985. Experimental infection of broiler chickens with rotavirus. Br. Vet. Jnl., 141, 69-73.

Mc Nulty, M.S., Curran, W.L., Todd, D., Mc Ferran, J.B. 1979. Detection of viruses in avian faeces by direct electron microscopy. Avian Path., 8, 239-247.

Mc Nulty, M.S., Allan, G.M., Connor, T.J., Mc Ferran, J.B., Mc Cracken, R.M. 1984. An entero-like virus associated with the runting syndrome in broiler chickens. Avian Path., 13, 429-439.

Page, R.K., Fletcher, O.J., Rowland, G.N., Gaudry, D., Villegas, P. 1982. Malabsorption syndrome in broiler chickens. Avian Dis., 26, 618-624.

Spackman, D., Gough, R.E., Collins, M.S., Lanning, D. 1984. Isolation of an enterovirus-like agent from the meconium of dead-in-shell chicken embryos. Vet. Rec., 114, 216-218.

Van der Heide, L., Lütticken, D., Horzinek, M. 1981. Isolation of avian reovirus as a possible etiologic agent of osteoporosis ("Brittle bone disease"; "Femoral head necrosis") in broiler chickens. Avian Dis., 25, 847-856.

FINDINGS IN HISTORY AND ETIOLOGY OF THE
STUNTING SYNDROME IN THE USA

D. Gaudry

Rhône Mérieux
69002 Lyon, France

ABSTRACT

A syndrome of broiler chickens characterised by stunted growth and abnormal feathering has been seen quite often in broiler farms of various countries. Scientists from Europe and North America have been looking for the origin of the problem which appears to be complex. From several experiments carried out at the laboratory and on the field, it appears that in the USA, some reovirus isolates should be incriminated in the etiology of the syndrome. American scientists as well are convinced that other factors including infectious agents are involved in the etiology of this syndrome, named Malabsorption Syndrome in the USA.

A runting syndrome of broiler chickens characterised by stunted growth, poor feathering and an increase in lameness has been described in 1978 (Kouwenhoven et al.). In affected flocks, 5-20% of the chicks exhibited growth retardation by one week of age; an increase in lameness and very poor feather development was apparent by two weeks of age. The most prevalent gross lesions were enlargement of the proventriculus and areas of necrosis, haemorrhages and catarrhal enteritis (Kouwenhoven et al., 1978).

In July 1979, L. van der Heide presented at the University of Georgia the results of his observations on the same subject and those obtained during his sabbatical year in Holland (1978-79). Two months later, at two-days interval, Lucien de Ruyttere from Belgium and David Kingston from Australia reported similar cases, the former suspecting a viral etiology, possibly a reticulo-endothelio-virus as responsible for the syndrome. This hypothesis was later abandoned.

L. de Ruyttere and D. Kingston visiting different farms in Georgia observed flocks revealing the same clinical signs which were treated for vitamins A and E deficiency.

From this time, more attention was given to this syndrome in the USA. Because of the variety of clinical signs and lesions, many names were given. Even a paper titled, "The disease of many faces and many names" was published (Weninger, 1982).

In fact, stunting was not the first thing that North American broiler growers noticed. As quite often the affected chicks display malpositioned or broken feathers on their wings which stand up like the propeller of a helicopter, this observation triggered off the name of "Helicopter disease".

Others were alerted by the paleness of the affected birds which resulted in the name of "Pale Bird Syndrome".

Then the laboratory diagnosticians tried to translate their pathological findings into more scientific names; due to the lesions of the proventriculus and referring to Kouwenhovens, publication, the name of "Infectious Proventriculitis" was used. Femoral Head Necrosis and Brittle Bones diseases were mentioned by others.

These different names pointed out the very confusing clinical picture for the diagnosticians who however all recognized a serious impairment of the digestive process and subsequently a malabsorption of all or some nutrients.

Once the malabsorption of nutrients had been clearly demonstrated (Page et al., 1982; Glass et al., 1973), all other symptoms and names may be easily conceived. The stunting is the result of an incomplete absorption of all nutrients (most importantly amino acids) which stops the development of the body. The poor feathering comes from the deficiency of methionine and vitamin A, while the lack of vitamins A and E are responsible for the paleness. The malabsorption of vitamin D, calcium, phosphorus and other minerals may explain brittle bones and several leg problems.

For that reason in the USA, the most common name used for this complex disease is "Malabsorption Syndrome" which points to the root of the problem and describes the malfunction of a process that is responsible for all the various side affects. Perhaps the word "infectious" should precede it, to signify the primary cause of the disorder. This primary cause, the absolute identity of the infectious agent or more probably, agents involved is not yet resolved.

In the USA, during the five past years scientists in Connecticut, Delaware and Georgia have been actively searching for the etiology of the Malabsorption Syndrome.

While Rotaviruses, Enteroviruses, Parvoviruses have been incriminated in Europe, Reoviruses might represent a piece of the puzzle for the American scientists.

Most probably the first work in the USA to look for a possible viral etiology was performed by the University of Georgia in February 1980. Virus isolations were attempted from intestinal homogenates and visceral organs of affected birds. Embryonated eggs from broiler breeders were initially used, then later on chicken kidney cell cultures (Page et al., 1982). Amongst revealed agents, reoviruses were predominant as expected. The real question was to determine the ability of these reoviruses to reproduce the syndrome.

During 1980-81, Dr K. Page dedicated a lot of this time on this subject with nonconvincing results. Many of the isolated strains did not seem to be pathogenic. Only some of them (CO8 and 81-5) were able to provoke some symptoms and lesions from the syndrome such as feather abnormalities, weight depression, undigested contents, etc. But none of these signs could be reproduced regularly in the inoculated birds.

At the end of 1981, no conclusion was still reached on the role of the reovirus in the Malabsorption Syndrome.

Whilst researchers in the laboratory were pursuing their efforts, another approach was taken by testing the influence of an adjuvanted killed vaccine produced from the CO8 strain on young broiler breeders known to reproduce the syndrome in the field. One-day old chickens were taken from the hatchery and brought to the laboratory; 50 of them were vaccinated by SC route, 0.2 ml/bird and 50 kept as control birds. After 8 weeks of observation, it was obvious that the vaccinated group was superior to the control group, having a better growth, size homogenicity, feathering and less lesions.

This trial had as consequence an increasing use of the vaccine in the field in Georgia and Alabama initially on one-day old broilers (1.6 million birds were vaccinated) and later on parent flocks to achieve the desired early protection of the progeny by parental antibodies. These experimental vaccinations on a large scale basis were criticized by some scientists who claimed that this was nonsense to use such a vaccine which was simply a viral arthritis (V.A.) vaccine.

Actually, all new reovirus isolates did cross react more or less with a specific antiserum to the viral arthritis 1133 strain. But if the 1133 V.A. vaccines were effective against the Malabsorption Syndrome, why so many cases of this syndrome were reported at this time from V.A. vaccinated birds? It may be suspected that the highly attenuated V.A. live vaccines were not immunogenic enough to protect the progeny of vaccinated breeders. Anyhow it was soon clearly demonstrated from the results obtained in the field as well as by challenge tests at the laboratory that the CO8 vaccine was a serious V.A. vaccine candidate.

During the time that this vaccine was tested in the field, more progress was made regarding the pathogenesis of the reoviruses suspected to be a cause of the Malabsorption Syndrome.

More highly pathogenic strains were isolated on chickens as 172 and 176 isolates. Foot-pad inoculation of one-day old broilers or leghorn origin chickens killed 80 to 100% of the birds in two to four days whilst oral inoculation was slightly less lethal with 60 to 100% mortality in four to five days (Hieronymus et al., 1983).

Other isolates were made from turkeys showing a variety of clinical signs, including high early mortality, stunted growth, poor feathering and diarrhoea (Goodwin et al., 1984). These isolates were lethal for young susceptible turkeys. Performance of 90,000 poults from non-vaccinated breeders were compared with the ones of 90,000 poults from breeders vaccinated with CO8 vaccine. The vaccine seems to have been highly beneficial, which let us suspect a common etiology (partially or totally) for the Malabsorption Syndrome of broilers and turkeys. The high pathogenicity of the 172 and 176 strains was of great help in the study of parameters to be considered for the reproduction of the malabsorption syndrome:

Age susceptibility:

Strains 172 and 176 when inoculated at 2-week old birds revealed little pathogenicity. This age resistance factor was previously reported (Sahu et al., 1975) using other isolates. It should be noted that 1133 V.A. strain is different from these strains by being capable to be still highly pathogenic for 10-week old chicks.

Genetic status of the bird:

Isolate 2177 was totally safe on SPAFAS one-day old chickens but creates lesions on other SPF chickens from another source.

Environment:

This parameter including flock management, food quality, other infectious agents interference is of most importance. It is also the one which

194

is the most difficult to handle.

In the USA, it is generally accepted that reovisuses are playing an effective role in the Malabsorption Syndrome in broilers as well as in young turkeys. With the development of killed vaccines from recently isolated reoviruses and the setting up of a more accurate vaccination program, viral arthritis and Malabsorption Syndrome are not at present a real problem in the USA. However, because Malabsorption Syndrome has been recognized as a transient syndrome varying with seasons and years, and has not been reported lately, it is difficult to make a clear cut statement about the benefit brought in the USA by the use of Malabsorption Syndrome vaccines. Because American scientists do consider that reovirus by itself is not the complete explanation of the Malabsorption Syndrome, they are paying great attention to the results obtained in Europe regarding this subject. Some are actively searching for other reasons than reovirus; possibilities of rotavirus involvement in this syndrome are presently under investigation (Yason, 1985).

REFERENCES

Glass, S.E., Naqi, S.A., Hall, C.F. and Kerr, K.M. 1973. Isolation and characterization of a virus associated with arthritis of chickens. Avian Diseases, 17, 415-525.
Goodwin, Mark A., Latimer, K.S., Nersessian, B.N. and Fletcher, O.J. 1984. Quantitation of Intestinal D-Xylose absorption in Normal and Reovirus-inoculated turkeys, Avian Diseases, 28, 959-967.
Hieronymus, D.R.K., Villegas, P. and Kleven, S.H. 1983. Characteristics and pathogenicity of two avian reoviruses isolated from chickens with leg problems. Avian Diseases, 27, 255-260.
Kouwenhoven, B., Vertommen, M. and Van Eck, J.H.H. 1978. Runting and leg weakness in broilers: Involvement of infectious factors. Vet. Sci. Commun. 2, 253-259.
Kouwenhoven, B., Davelaar, F.G. and Van Walsum, J. 1978. Infectious proventriculitis causing runting in broilers. Avian Pathol. 7, 183-187.
Page, R.K. and Fletcher, O.J. 1982. Malabsorption syndrome in broiler chickens. Avian Diseases, 26, 618-624.
Page, R.K., Fletcher, O.J., Rowland, G.N., Gaudry, D. and Villegas, P. 1982. Case Report. Malabsorption Syndrome in broiler chickens. Avian Diseases, 26, 618-624.
Sahu, S.P. and Olson, N.O. 1975. Comparison of the characteristics of avian reoviruses isolated from the digestive and respiratory tract, with viruses isolated from the synovia. Am. J. Vet. Res. 36, 847-850.
Weninger, O. 1982. The disease of many faces (... & many names). Shaver Focus, 11, 4.
Yason, C. 1985. Infecciones causadas por rotavirus en pollos y pavos, IX Congreso Latino Americano de Avicultura, Acapulco.

RECENT ADVANCES IN ENTEROVIRUS INFECTIONS OF BIRDS

J. B. McFerran and M. S. McNulty

Veterinary Research Laboratories
Stormont, Belfast BT4 3SD.
Northern Ireland

ABSTRACT

A newly recognised enterovirus isolated in Japan, avian nephritis virus (ANV), has been shown to be widely distributed in birds in Northern Ireland and also in some European SPF flocks. Antibody to this virus is also prevalent in turkey but not duck flocks. An enterovirus-like particle (ELP) associated with runting and diarrhoea has been shown to be serologically identical to ANV, but different biologically. At least one other ELP of fowl and two turkey ELPs exist but have not yet been compared or fully characterised.

INTRODUCTION

Until recently the only avian enteroviruses recognised were the avian encephalomyelitis and duck virus hepatitis viruses. However, in recent years a number of new members have been recognised. This review will deal mainly with these newly recognised viruses.

The general properties of enteroviruses are given in table 1.

TABLE 1   General properties of Enteroviruses

Nucleic acid		RNA
Morphology		
	Size	28 ± 3 nm
	Shape	Spherical. No obvious structure
	Envelope	None
Stability		
	Resistant to	Chloroform
		pH3

All apparently have their main site of replication the intestine and more particularly the villous epithelial cells of the small intestine. However many have predeliction sites elsewhere and are associated with clinical illness involving these sites. Thus the poliomyelitis viruses

of man and the avian encephalomyelitis virus invade the central nervous
system.   Some human Coxsackie viruses cause lesions in the heart and the
pancreas.   Avian nephritis virus affects the kidneys and duck virus
hepatitis virus produces liver lesions.   In vitro growth is very
variable - some of the bovine enteroviruses grow in a wide variety of
cells, others e.g. the human and porcine enteroviruses grow in a restricted
number of cells and many of the avian members grow poorly or not at all in
cell culture.   The main property separating the enteroviruses from other
members of the Picornaviridae is pH3 stability.

The currently recognised members of the group are listed in table 2.

TABLE 2   Avian enteroviruses

Host Species	Virus designation		Reference
Fowl	Avian encephalomyelitis	(AE)	Butterfield et al., 1969
	Avian nephritis	(AN)	Yamaguchi et al., 1979
	Enterovirus-like particles	(ELPs)	Spackman et al., 1984
	Enterovirus-like particles	(ELPs)	McNulty et al., 1984a
	Enterovirus-like particles	(ELPs)	McNulty. Unpublished
Duck	Duck virus hepatitis	1 (DVH1)	Tauraso et al., 1969
	Duck virus hepatitis	2 (DVH2)	Asplin,1965; Gough et al. 1985
	Duck virus hepatitis	3 (DVH3)	Haider and Calnek, 1979
Turkey	Avian encephalomyelitis	(AE)	Deshmukh et al., 1973
	Enterovirus-like particles	(ELPs)	Macdonald et al., 1982
	Enterovirus-like particles	(ELPs)	McNulty. Unpublished

It should be noted that no member has been fully characterised and
in some the evidence that they are enteroviruses is only tenuous.   It
should be noted that duck virus hepatitis type 2 has now been shown to be
an astrovirus (Gough et al.,1985).

This communication deals primarily with the newly recognised members
of this group.

AVIAN NEPHRITIS

During studies on 2 broiler flocks in Japan, 7 isolates were made
from healthy 1 week old chickens.   All proved to be the same serotype and
one, G-4260, was studied (Yamaguchi et al., 1979).   This virus grew in

the cytoplasm with crystals of 30 nm hexagonal particles, was stable to treatment with organic solvents and trypsin and to pH3, was not inactivated by freezing and thawing or sonication. It passed a 50 nm filter and was not inactivated by IUDR. It caused an enterovirus-like cytopathic effect in chick kidney cell cultures and 2.4 nm diameter plaques, which were enhanced by the addition of diethylaminoethyl dextran. Maximum titres in CK cells occurred after 24 hours. Antiserum to this virus did not neutralise AE virus.

Following intraperitoneal (I/P) inoculation with AN virus, no clinical signs were seen in day old chicks, but a slower growth rate was found. Virus was widely distributed, with maximum titres in the kidneys and jejunum and lower titres in the bursa of Fabricus, spleen and liver (Imada et al., 1979) and there were focal lesions in the kidney cortex (Maeda et al., 1979). Work by the same group showed that chickens could be infected by a variety of routes. Oral inoculation was best, producing gross lesions in the kidney with a microscopic nephritis. Only birds infected 1 and 14 days of age developed gross lesions, 28 day old birds developed nephritis. At 58 and 300 days pi all were infected. The chick infective dose fifty was calculated to be between $10^{0.9}$ and $10^{1.7}$ pfus (Imada et al., 1981). The virus apparently has no effect on egg production or egg quality   (Imada et al., 1983).

Antibody to AN virus was widely distributed in Japanese layer and broiler flocks after 1973 but there was no evidence in sera collected in 1965 or 1972 (Imada et al., 1980). A survey of flocks in Northern Ireland indicated that infection with AN has been widespread in fowl flocks since 1975. It is also widely distributed in turkey flocks. No antibody was detected in duck sera (Connor et al., 1985). It should be noted that antibody to AN was also detected in a number of SPF flocks, including SPF flocks selling eggs commercially.

FOWL ENTEROVIRUS-LIKE PARTICLES (ELPs)

During studies of both enteritis and runting in broilers, small round virus-like particles of around 30 nm diameter were commonly seen during the first week of life. There is no direct evidence that these viruses are egg transmitted, although the frequency in which they appear in faeces of day old chicks suggest they are. When faeces containing ELPs were inoculated into day old broilers diarrhoea and interference with growth were observed (McFerran et al., 1983, 1984; McNulty et al., 1984a). This virus grows in the cytoplasm of the villous epithelium cells of the small intestine. Although the virus grows in the cytoplasm of chick kidney cells and chick embryo liver cells it cannot be serially passaged (McNulty et al., 1984a). A second ELP virus has been isolated from broilers aged 27 days. This virus is not antigenically related to ELPs or to AE virus and it can be serially passaged in eggs by CAM inoculation (McNulty, unpublished).

However, there is direct evidence that some ELPs are egg transmitted with the isolation of an ELP from the meconium of dead-in-shell chicken embryos (Spackman et al., 1984). This virus was pH3, chloroform and trypsin stable. It was partially inactivated by 56°C and withstood 50°C. It was not related to duck virus hepatitis or avian encephalomyelitis virus, but there is no information on its relationship to the Northern Ireland serotypes.

ANTIGENIC RELATIONSHIPS BETWEEN SOME AVIAN ENTEROVIRUSES

Cross immunofluorescence and serum neutralisation tests between AE, AN, DVH and the ELP described by McNulty et al. (1984a) demonstrated that AE, AN and DVH viruses were not related to each other. However, it appeared that AN virus and ELPs are antigenically identical. However, when inoculated orally AE, AN and DVH did not cause any significant growth retardation, whereas ELPs caused a 40% weight reduction at 2 weeks (McFerran et al., 1985).

TURKEY ENTEROVIRUS-LIKE VIRUSES

McNulty et al. (1979) described ELPs in the faeces of turkeys. Subsequently we have found ELPs on a number of times in the faeces of runted turkeys, turkeys with diarrhoea and also from normal turkeys. These viruses have been seen in day old turkeys, suggesting egg transmission.

Workers in Lasswade, Scotland isolated an ELP from a turkey with hepatic necrosis. This virus grows in embryonated eggs following yolk sac inoculation. Following intraperitoneal or yolk sac inoculation of two day old turkeys no illness was produced but hepatic lesions were seen on autopsy (Macdonald et al., 1982). It is suggested that this virus is the cause of turkey virus hepatitis.

More recently French workers have found ELPs in the faeces of 15 day-

6 week old turkeys suffering from respiratory or digestive problems (Andral and Toquin, 1984). These could be grown in embryonated eggs and it was possible to distinguish 2 strains. There is no record of any comparison between the French, Scottish or Northern Irish strains, or between the ELPs of turkeys and fowl.

LONGITUDINAL STUDIES IN BROILER FLOCKS

When both normal and runted flocks are sampled at weekly or twice weekly intervals certain patterns of virus excretion appear common (McFerran et al., 1983, 1984). Using chick embryo liver cells reoviruses are the main isolates from faeces during the first weeks of life. Although some isolates may be made during the first few days of life, the main excretion occurs from 7-21 days of age. There is sometimes another wave of excretion around 42-48 days. Then adenovirus excretion takes over and continues until the flock is slaughtered between 42 and 70 days. Occasionally adenoviruses are excreted in the first week of life. There may be 4 or more reovirus or adenovirus serotypes present in a large broiler flock.

If direct electron microscopic (EM) examination (McNulty et al., 1979) of faeces is used a different picture emerges. It is rare to see adenoviruses or reoviruses by direct EM. ELPs type 1 are present from day old onwards until about 10 days. A second burst of ELPs are sometimes seen around 25-32 days and these are ELP type 2. Rotaviruses appear around 15 days (although sometimes are present earlier). In large flocks, rotaviruses are almost continually present until slaughter. Usually 3 or 4 serogroups of rotavirus are present (McNulty et al. 1984b). Other viruses such as astroviruses or caliciviruses are occasionally present.

IMPORTANCE OF THESE ENTEROVIRUSES

There is no doubt that some enteroviruses, such as poliomyelitis in man and avian encephalomyelitis are important pathogens. However, there are very many enteroviruses recognised which are either non-pathogenic or whose role as pathogens are ill-defined.

Enteroviruses are widely distributed. Thus, there are at least 63 human serotypes. At present there are at least 3 fowl, 2 duck and 2 turkey enteroviruses. But by analogy with mammals there is no reason to believe that further serotypes will not be discovered. The problem is that whilst they are relatively easy to recognise in faeces using direct electron microscopic examination, they are very difficult to grow in vitro. Immunofluorescence can help by allowing the recognition of viruses which grow, even for only 1 passage, in cell culture producing no or a poor cytopathic effect. However, this technique probably only detects group antigen and there may be a number of different serotypes, based on serum neutralisation which will go undetected. In addition as already described viruses identical by serological methods may show marked biological differences.

The importance of these ELPs in the aetiology of runting is debatable. They do produce a failure of day old chicks to show a normal growth curve for 2-3 weeks in addition to diarrhoea and some retardation of feather development. But the effect is not permanent, although this simply may be due to too few birds being used, as permanently affected birds (the runts) may only be 1% of an infected flock. ELPs are present in the embryonated egg and during the first week of life at a time when presumably the pathological processes associated with runting are in operation. This would also apply to reoviruses, but we have been unable to reproduce the same pattern with purified reoviruses. It should be noted that faeces preparations of reoviruses made from runting cases were contaminated with ELPs but would not have been detected unless examined using the electron microscope. Rotaviruses also cause a less severe failure to grow, associated with a diarrhoea. But in the runted flocks we have studied, rotaviruses are not usually present until 15 days, by which time the affected flocks are beginning to recover.

Therefore, in summary, workers should be aware that these viruses are present. They may well avoid detection by normal virological techniques and at present the importance of some of the more recently recognised members is yet to be established. In particular, the fact that they are present in some SPF flocks and are probably egg transmitted, has implications for both research workers and vaccine manufacturers. Furthermore, workers using faeces suspensions or low passage virus pools should check to see if the preparations are free from unsuspected ELPs.

REFERENCES

Andral, B. and Toquin, D. 1984. Observations et isolements de pseudopicornavirus a partir de dindonneaux malades. Avian Pathology 13, 377-388.

Asplin, F.D. 1965. Duck hepatitis: vaccination against two serological
    types. The Veterinary Record 77, 1529-1530.
Butterfield, W.K. Luginbuhl, R.E. and Helmboldt, C.F. 1969.
    Characterization of avian encephalomyelitis virus (an avian
    enterovirus). Avian Diseases, 13, 363-378.
Connor, T.J., McNeilly, F. and McFerran, J.B. 1985. A serological survey
    for antibody to avian nephritis virus in birds in Northern
    Ireland. In preparation.
Deshmukh, D.R., Hohlstein, W.M., McDowell, J.R. and Pomeroy, B.S. 1971.
    Prevalence of avian encephalomyelitis in turkey breeder flocks.
    American Journal of Veterinary Research, 32, 1263-1267.
Gough, R.E., Collins, M.S., Borland, E.D. and Keymer, I.F. 1984.
    Astrovirus-like particles associated with hepatitis in ducklings.
    The Veterinary Record, 144, 279.
Haider, S.A. and Calnek, B.W. 1979. In vitro isolation, propagation and
    characterization of duck hepatitis virus type III. Avian Diseases,
    23, 715-729.
Imada, T., Yamaguchi, S. and Kawamura, H. 1979. Pathogenicity for baby
    chicks of the G-4260 strain of picornavirus 'Avian Nephritis Virus'.
    Avian Diseases, 23, 582-588.
Imada, T., Yamaguchi, S., Miura, N. and Kawamura, H. 1980. Antibody
    survey against avian nephritis virus among chickens in Japan.
    National Institute of Animal Health Quarterly, Japan. 20, 79-80.
Imada, T., Taniguchi, T., Yamaguchi, S., Minetoma, T., Maeda, M. and
    Kawamura, H. 1981. Susceptibility of chickens to avian nephritis
    virus at various inoculation routes and ages. Avian Diseases. 25,
    294-302.
Imada, T., Maeda, M., Furuta, K., Yamaguchi, S. and Kawamura, H. 1983.
    Pathogenesis and distribution of avian nephritis (G-4260 strain)
    in inoculated laying hens. National Institute of Animal Health
    Quarterly, Japan 23, 43-48.
McDonald, J.W., Randall, C.J. and Dagless, M.D. 1982. Picorna-like virus
    causing hepatitis and panoreatitis in turkeys. The Veterinary
    Record, 111, 323.
McFerran, J.B., McNulty, M.S., McCracken, R.M. and Greene, J. 1983.
    Enteritis and associated problems. In 'Disease prevention and
    control in poultry production' pp 129-140. The Post-Graduate
    Committee in Veterinary Medicine, University of Sydney, Sydney,
    Australia.
McFerran, J.B., Connor, T.J., McNulty, M.S. and McCracken, R.M. 1984.
    Infectious runting. 'Proc. 33rd Western Poultry Disease Conference'
    pp 73-77 University of California, Davis, USA.
McFerran, J.B. Connor, T.J. and McNeilly, F. 1985. Studies on some
    avian enteroviruses. In preparation.
McNulty, M.S., Todd, D., Allan, G.M., McFerran, J.B. and Greene, J.A.
    1984b. Epidemiology of rotavirus infection in broiler chickens:
    recognition of four serogroups. Archives of Virology, 81, 113-121.
McNulty, M.S., Allan, G.M., Connor, T.J., McFerran, J.B. and McCracken R.M.
    1984a. An entero-like virus associated with the runting syndrome in
    broiler chickens. Avian Pathology, 13, 429-439.
McNulty, M.S., Curran, W.L., Todd, D. and McFerran, J.B. 1979.
    Detection of viruses on avian faeces by direct electron microscopy.
    Avian Pathology, 8, 239-247.
Maeda, M., Imada, T., Taniguchi, T. and Horiuchi, T. 1979. Pathological
    changes in chicks inoculated with picorna virus 'Avian Nephritis
    Virus'. Avian Diseases, 23, 589-596.

Spackman, D., Gough, R.C., Collins, M.S. and Lanning, D. 1984. Isolation
    of an enterovirus-like agent from the meconium of dead-in-shell
    chicken embryos. The Veterinary Record, 144, 216-218.
Tauraso, N.M., Coghill, C.E., and Klutch, M.J. 1969. Properties of the
    attenuated vaccine strain of duck hepatitis virus. Avian Diseases 13,
    321-329.
Yamaguchi, S. Imada, T. and Kawamura, H. 1979. Characterization of
    picornavirus isolated from broiler chicks. Avian Diseases, 23,
    571-581.

AVIAN INFECTIOUS ANAEMIA

CAUSED BY CHICKEN ANAEMIA AGENT (CAA)

V. v. Bülow*, B. Fuchs*, R. Rudolph**

Free University Berlin
*Institute of Poultry Diseases
**Institute of Veterinary Pathology
D-1000 Berlin 33 (West), Germany

ABSTRACT

Chicken anaemia agent (CAA) has been studied in vivo and in vitro. Avian infectious anaemia (AIA) was considerably aggravated in chicks dually infected at day-old with CAA and virulent Marek's disease virus (MDV), infectious bursal disease virus (IBDV), or reticuloendotheliosis virus (REV). CAA-induced gross and histological lesions were characterized by panmyelophthisis and generalized lymphoid atrophy, and resembled those of the syndrome of anaemia, panmyelopathy and haemorrhagic diathesis occurring in the field. Circumstantial evidence suggested that CAA is also causing a severe immunodepression in neonatally infected chicks.

CAA replicates in cultured cells of the MDCC-MSB1 lymphoblastoid cell line. Cytopathic effects occurred by 30 hours postinoculation (p.i.) and were characterized by enlargement and subsequent destruction of cells. Infected MSB1 cells have been found to be suitable at 34 to 44 hours p.i. for indirect immunofluorescence tests to detect intranuclear CAA antigens or anti-CAA antibody, respectively.

INTRODUCTION

Chicken anaemia agent (CAA) is the causative agent of avian infectious anaemia and was first isolated by Yuasa et al. (1979). In SPF chicks neonatally infected by intramuscular inoculation, CAA causes an anaemia and pancytopenia between 8 and 20 days p.i. with a maximum between 14 and 16 days. Principal gross lesions consist in a more or less complete atrophy of bone marrow and thymus. Mortality of singly CAA-infected chicks is rather low. Reconvalescence starts as early as 16 to 18 days p.i. and usually is complete by 24 to 32 days p.i. (Yuasa et al., 1979; Taniguchi et al., 1983). Age-resistance against avian infectious anaemia develops during the first 7 days of life and is complete by 14 days. However, if day-old chicks are infected with infectious bursal disease virus (IBDV), age-resistance against anaemia is delayed by 2 to 3 weeks (Yuasa et al., 1980b). Maternal antibodies have been found to confer protection against infectious anaemia (Yuasa et al., 1980b). Single CAA infection of day-old chicks by contact does not cause anaemia. However, dual infection by contact with IBDV and CAA has been found to cause infectious anaemia with high mortality (Yuasa et al.,

1980b). This may have important implications with regard to the pathogenesis of CAA infection in the field. CAA can also be vertically transmitted. Transmission of CAA has been detected by eggs laid between 8 and 14 days after experimental infection of hens (Yuasa and Yoshida, 1983).

Highest titres of CAA have been detected in liver, thymus and spleen of neonatally infected chickens at 7 and 14 days p.i., and viraemia occurs from 1 to 7 days p.i. with a peak at 7 days. The agent persists in several tissues and in intestinal contents for at least 7 weeks but may be eliminated more rapidly in birds infected at 28 or 42 days of age (Yuasa et al., 1983a). Chicken liver is the preferred source of CAA for attempts of agent isolation. According to investigations of Yuasa et al. (1983b) and to studies in our laboratory, CAA is wide-spread in our chicken populations and may be considered as an ubiquitous infectious agent which may well play an important part in a number of mixed infections occurring in the field.

CAA can be propagated and assayed in cultures of the MDCC-MSB1 lymphoblastoid cell line whereas many other types and lines of cultured avian cells have been found to be unsuitable for CAA replication (Yuasa, 1983). Thus it became possible to employ cell cultures for neutralization tests (Yuasa et al., 1983a) which formerly could only be performed in chickens (Yuasa et al., 1980a).

Physicochemical properties of CAA indicate that this agent is likely to be a small virus like parvoviruses, but the true nature of CAA has not yet been identified. CAA is resistant to ether and chloroform, heat-resistant (1 hour at 70°C), acid-resistant (pH 3 for 3 hours), and it passes filter membranes with a 25 nm pore size (Yuasa et al., 1979).

The purpose of recent studies reported in this paper was to gain further knowledge about properties of CAA in vitro and in vivo with special reference to its possible importance in the field. Experimental methods and results will be described in more detail in two papers which are to be published by the end of this year (Bülow et al., 1985a,b).

EXPERIMENTS AND RESULTS

Growth and assay of CAA in MDCC-MSB1 cell cultures

CAA strains Gifu-1 (Yuasa et al., 1979) and Cux-1 (Bülow et al., 1983) were employed throughout the experiments.

Assay of CAA infectivity in MSB1 cell cultures turned out to be an unusually lengthy procedure, for several reasons. In our hands, CAA titres in culture supernatants increase by only 10-fold or little more within 3 to 4 days p.i., although Yuasa (1983) achieved a 100-fold multiplication in his subline of MSB1 cells. In several instances, susceptibility of continuously cultured MSB1 cells to CAA decreased within 4 to 12 weeks (including sub-cultures every 3 to 4 days), for unknown reasons. Minor CAA-induced cyto-pathic effects (CPE) cannot readily be recognized because MSB1 cells are growing in suspension, and low numbers of infected cells are rapidly over-grown by the non-infected cells. Inoculated cells have therefore to be sub-cultured every 3 to 4 days until a CPE can clearly be recognized and cells discontinue to multiply. As a result, a complete titration requires at least 6 to 8 subcultures, i.e. 4 to 5 weeks.

An immediate CPE could be achieved by inoculating cell cultures with CAA at a multiplicity of at least 5 $TCID_{50}$ per cell. In sufficiently infec-ted cultures, most cells become considerably swollen by 30 hours p.i., and cell destruction begins at 34 hours p.i. increasing during the following 24 hours. Maximal cell-associated infectivity between 24 and 48 hours p.i. hardly exceeded about 10 $TCID_{50}$ per cultured cell. Small granula of intra-nuclear CAA antigen could be demonstrated by indirect immunofluorescence assays as early as 34 hours p.i. and thereafter in at least 50% of the swollen MSB1 cells. The indirect fluorescent antibody (FA) test turned out to be a sensitive and rapid method for detecting anti-CAA antibody in chicken serum or in egg yolk. In quantitative antibody assays, SN tests were slightly more sensitive than FA tests.

A variety of other avian cell lines has been tested for susceptibility to CAA infection. These included producer cell lines MDCC-CU12, CU25 and CU40; non-producer cell lines MDCC-HP1, HP2, HP3, HP10, RP1, and a different subline of MDCC-MSB1; lines LLCC-HP45, HP46, HP50, HP73 and HP76. All these cell lines proved to be resistant to CAA infection. This may also suggest that there is no significant helper effect of MDV or MDV genome on CAA replication.

Effects of CAA infection in singly inoculated chicks

Avian infectious anaemia was studied in chicks neonatally inoculated i.m. with CAA strains Gifu-1 or Cux-1, or with a field isolate of CAA de-signated K85. Materials employed were either cell-free liver homogenate from CAA-infected chickens at 10 to 14 days p.i., or supernatants of CAA-infected MSB1 cell cultures. The dose per chicken varied between 6×10^4 to 2×10^5 $TCID_{50}$. Anaemia developed within 14 days p.i. and was associated with marked atrophy of the bone marrow, almost complete regression of the

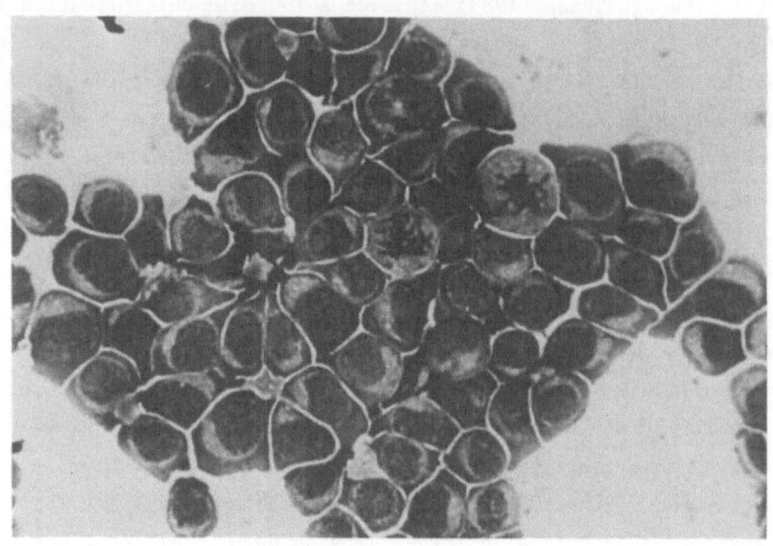

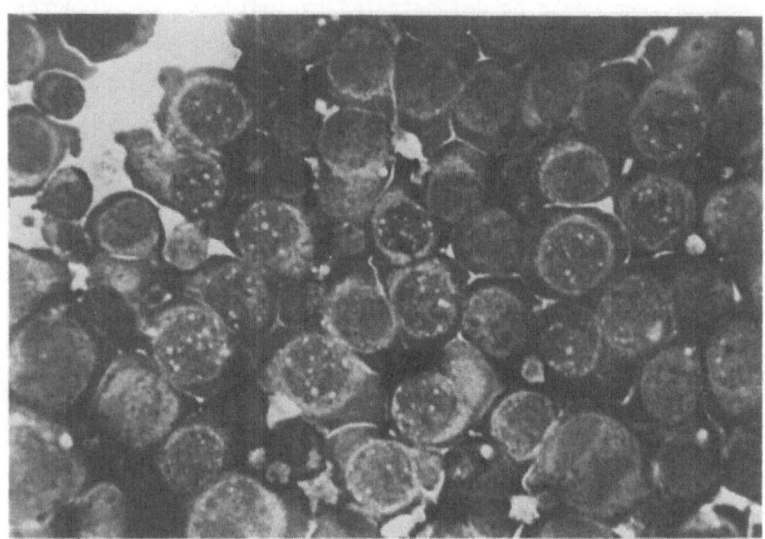

Fig. 1   Morphological changes of cultured MSB1 cells caused by
chicken anaemia agent (CAA) within 32 hours p.i. (below), compared
with uninfected controls (above). (May-Grünwald and Giemsa, x 190).

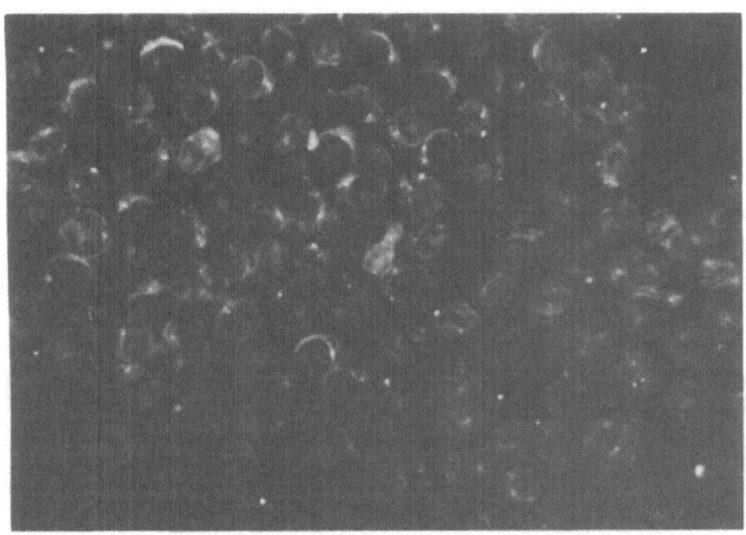

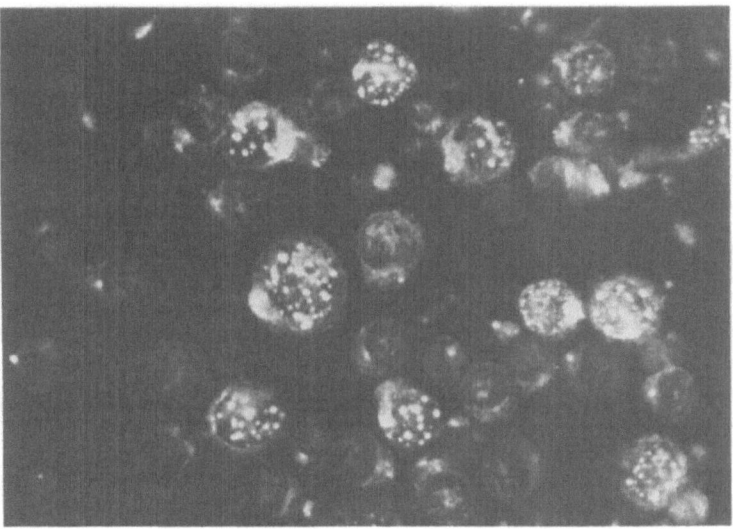

Fig. 2   Intranuclear fluorescent antigen in cultured MSB1 cells at 36 hours after infection with chicken anaemia agent (below), compared with uninfected negative controls (above). (Indirect immunofluorescence, x 190).

thymus, and bursal atrophy. Mortality occurring between 13 and 18 days p.i. did never exceed 30%. Susceptibility to secondary bacterial infections was obviously increased, suggesting the presence of CAA-induced immunosuppression.

Histological examination of various tissues largely confirmed the results of Taniguchi et al. (1983). Histopathological alterations in anaemic chicks at 14 days p.i. could be characterized as panmyelophthisis and generalized lymphoid atrophy involving all haematopoietic and lymphoid tissues. The most striking lesion was panmyelophthisis seen in the bone marrow, i.e. atrophy and aplasia, with edema, in some cases necrosis of cell foci, and proliferation of stroma. Thymus cortex and medulla were equally atrophic, with hydropic degeneration of residual cells and occasional necrotic foci. Lesions in the bursa of Fabricius were atrophy and necrosis of follicles, infolded epithelium, hydropic epithelial degeneration, and proliferation of stroma tissue. Atrophy of lymphoid tissue, sometimes necrosis involving lymphoid follicles and Schweiger-Seidel sheaths, and some haemorrhages were present in the spleen. In caecal tonsils, liver, kidney, and proventriculus, lymphoid foci were depleted of cells, smaller and less dense than those in intact birds.

Dual infection of chicks with CAA and immunosupressive viruses

A particular field isolate of classical Marek's disease virus (MDV) causing an early mortality syndrome with lesions like those of infectious anaemia had been found to be contaminated with CAA, which was subsequently designated Cux-1 strain (Bülow et al., 1983). For this and other reasons we became especially interested in the effects of dual infection of day-old chickens with MDV, IBDV, or reticuloendotheliosis virus (REV). Viruses used in dual inoculations included the HPRS-16 and HPRS-B14 strains of virulent MDV, the HPRS-24 strain of non-oncogenic MDV, the Cu-1 strain of pathogenic IBDV, and the REV-C strain of non-transforming REV. All these viruses, except for the HPRS-24 strain of MDV are known to cause immunosuppression in chicks but by different mechanisms. The HPRS-24 strain of MDV turned out not to have any obvious effect in dual infections with CAA.

Dual infection of day-old chickens with CAA and either virulent MDV, IBDV or REV invariably resulted in a considerable aggravation of infectious anaemia. That included an increase of mortality up to 100% between 10 and 14 days p.i., enhancement of CAA-induced lesions, higher frequency of haemorrhages, and increased susceptibility to bacterial infections. Furthermore, it was obvious that protective effects of anti-CAA maternal antibody could become ineffective or were reduced in dually infected birds. Reconvalescence of surviving dually infected anaemic chicks was retarded as indicated by a longer persistence of anaemia and of histological lesions. The principal results of these experiments are summarized in Table 1.

TABLE 1   Avian infectious anaemia (AIA) in chickens singly inoculated with chicken anaemia agent (CAA), or dually inoculated with Marek's disease virus (MDV), infectious bursal disease virus (IBDV), or reticuloendotheliosis virus (REV).

Exp.[a]	Inoculation 1	Inoculation 2	Mortality	Total incidence of AIA (anaemia + mortality)[b]	
1A	CAA	–	0%	100%	(HT 17.8%)[c]
	CAA	MDV	42%*	92%	(HT 15.0%)
1B	CAA	–	0%	13%	(HT 21.9%)
	CAA	MDV	87%**	87%**	(HT 12.3%)
2A	CAA	–	20%	80%	(HT 18.5%)
	CAA	IBDV	67%*	95%	(HT 14.0%)
2B	CAA	–	25%	33%	(HT 17.6%)
	CAA	IBDV	40%	80%*	(HT 14.8%)
3A	CAA	–	7%	89%	(HT 19.6%)
	CAA	REV	100%**	100%	(HT 12.6%)
3B	CAA	–	30%	60%	(HT 13.5%)
	CAA	REV	85%*	92%	(HT 16.0%)
4	CAA	–	0%	0%	–
	CAA	MDV	0%	29%*	(HT 25.5%)
	CAA	IBDV	13%	17%	(HT 25.4%)

[a]A, no anti-CAA antibody detected in the parent flocks; B, parent flock with anti-CAA antibody; exp. 4, high levels of anti-CAA maternal antibody.

[b]Occasional bone marrow atrophy in non-anaemic chicks has been disregarded in these data.

[c]HT = haematokrit, mean values of anaemic chicks at 14 days p.i.; chicks with HT values of up to 27% were considered anaemic; HT values of non-anaemic chicks were in the range of 34%.

* $p < 0.05$, ** $p < 0.01$, statistically significant differences between singly and dually infected groups of chickens.

DISCUSSION AND CONCLUSIONS

Experimental results are strongly suggesting that CAA may well play an important role in the etiology of certain multifactorial diseases occurring among young chickens in the field. The generalized lymphoid atrophy seen in CAA-infected birds and their increased susceptibility to unintentional bacterial infection may be considered as indicative of immunosuppressive effects of CAA infection. On the other hand, the synergistic effects of MDV, IBDV or REV on CAA infection are probably due to immunosuppressive effects of those three virus species. A variety of other factors with similar effects on CAA pathogenicity are not unlikely to occur in the natural environment of young chickens.

There was a striking similarity between the condition seen in dually infected chickens and the syndrome of panmyelopathy, anaemia, haemorrhagic diathesis and dermatitis affecting young chicks, especially broiler chicks, in the field. This syndrome has been reported by many authors during the past 12 years (Dorn et al., 1981; Engström and Luthman, 1984; Fadly and Winterfield, 1973; Hoffmann and Dorn, 1978; Hoffmann et al., 1973 & 1975; Köhler and Hromatka-Vasicek, 1974; Randall et al., 1984; Rosenberger et al., 1975). Especially, the histological lesions described by Dorn et al. (1981) and Hoffmann et al. (1975) largely resemble the lesions seen in our dually infected chicks. Inclusion body hepatitis, sometimes also associated with this syndrome, can easily be explained by additional infection with adenoviruses. We have seen that experimental adenovirus- or reovirus-induced hepatitis can well occur together with CAA-induced infectious anaemia, however there is obviously no synergistic effect between these viruses and CAA.

The difficulties in the past to reproduce the naturally occurring syndrome by experimental infection can largely be explained now. Environmental factors aggravating the effects of CAA infection are usually difficult to identify. It may therefore be of some help in conducting future experiments to know that it may be possible to overcome natural resistance of chicks by dual infection with the material to be assayed for the presence of CAA and with an immunosuppressive virus, such as IBDV, REV, or virulent MDV. On the other hand, many in vivo experiments can now be omitted since the indirect FA test provides a most useful tool for identifying suspected CAA isolates as well as for detecting anti-CAA antibody.

REFERENCES

Bülow, V.v., Fuchs, B., Vielitz, E. and Landgraf, H. 1983. Frühsterblich-keitssyndrom bei Küken nach Doppelinfektion mit dem Virus der Marek-schen Krankheit (MDV) und einem Anämie-Erreger (CAA). Zbl. Vet. Med. B, 30, 742-750.

Bülow, V.v., Fuchs, B. and Bertram, M. 1985a. Untersuchungen über den Erre-ger der infektiösen Anämie bei Hühnerküken (CAA) in vitro: Vermehrung, Titration, Serumneutralisationstest und indirekter Immunfluoreszenz-test. Zbl. Vet. Med. B (in press).

Bülow, V.v., Rudolph, R. and Fuchs, B. 1985b. Erhöhte Pathogenität des Er-regers einer infektiösen Anämie bei Hühnerküken (CAA) bei simultaner Infektion mit dem Virus der Marekschen Krankheit (MDV), Bursitisvirus (IBDV) oder Reticuloendotheliosevirus (REV). Zbl. Vet. Med. B (in press).

Dorn, P., Weikel, J. and Wessling, E. 1981. Anämie, Rückbildung der lympha-tischen Organe und Dermatitis - Beobachtungen zu einem neuen Krank-heitsbild in der Geflügelmast. Dtsch. Tierärztl. Wschr., 88, 313-315.

Engström, B.E. and Luthman, M. 1984. Blue wing disease of chickens: Signs, pathology and natural transmission. Avian Pathol., 13, 1-12.

Fadly, A.M. and Winterfield, R.W. 1973. Isolation and some characteristics of an agent associated with inclusion body hepatitis, hemorrhages, and aplastic anemia in chickens. Avian Dis., 17, 182-193.

Hoffmann, R. and Dorn, P. 1978. Histological development of lesions in the bursa of Fabricius of chickens with inclusion body hepatitis. Avian Dis., 22, 266-272.

Hoffmann, R., Dorn, P. and Dangschat, H. 1973. Ein neues durch Panmyelopa-thie, Anämie und hämorrhagische Diathese gekennzeichnetes Syndrom beim Huhn. Zbl. Vet. Med. B, 20, 741-746.

Hoffmann, R., Wessling, E., Dorn, P. and Dangschat, H. 1975. Lesions in chickens with spontaneous or experimental infectious hepato-myelopoie-tic disease. Avian Dis., 19, 224-236.

Köhler, H. and Hromatka-Vasicek, L. 1974. Einschlußkörper-Hepatitis bei Broilern in Österreich. Wien. Tierärztl. Mschr., 61, 90-95.

Randall, C.J., Miller, W.G., Wallis, A.S. and Kirkpatrick, K.S. 1984. Multiple infections in young broilers. Vet. Rec., 114, 270-271.

Rosenberger, J.K., Klopp, S., Eckroade, R.J. and Krauss, W.C. 1975. The role of infectious bursal agent and several avian adenoviruses in the hemorrhagic-aplastic-anemia syndrome and gangrenous dermatitis. Avian Dis., 19, 717-729.

Taniguchi, T., Yuasa, N., Maeda, M. and Horiuchi, T. 1983. Chronological observations on hemato-pathological changes in chicks inoculated with chicken anemia agent. Natl. Inst. Anim. Health Quart., 23, 1-12.

Yuasa, N. 1983. Propagation and infectivity titration of the Gifu-1 strain of chicken anemia agent in a cell line (MDCC-MSB1) derived from Marek's disease lymphoma. Natl. Inst. Anim. Health Quart., 23, 13-30.

Yuasa, N. and Yoshida, I. 1983. Experimental egg transmission of chicken anemia agent. Natl. Inst. Anim. Health Quart., 23, 99-100.

Yuasa, N., Taniguchi, T. and Yoshida, I. 1979. Isolation and some characte-ristics of an agent inducing anemia in chicks. Avian Dis., 23, 366-385.

Yuasa, N., Noguchi, T., Furata, K. and Yoshida, I. 1980a. Maternal antibody and its effect on the susceptibility of chicks to chicken anemia agent. Avian Dis., 24, 197-201.

Yuasa, N., Taniguchi, T., Noguchi, T. and Yoshida, I. 1980b. Effect of in-fectious bursal disease virus infection of chickens on anemia by chicken anemia agent. Avian Dis., 24, 202-209.

Yuasa, N., Taniguchi, T., Imada, T. and Hihara, H. 1983a. Distribution of chicken anemia agent (CAA) and detection of neutralizing antibody in chicks experimentally inoculated with CAA. Natl. Inst. Anim. Health Quart., 23, 78-81.

Yuasa, N., Taniguchi, T., Goda, M., Shibatani, M., Imada, T. and Hihara, H. 1983b. Isolation of chicken anemia agent with MDCC-MSB1 cells from chickens in the field. Natl. Inst. Anim. Health Quart., 23, 75-77.

RECENT ADVANCES IN DUCK VIRAL HEPATITIS

H. Farmer*†, W.S.K. Chalmers**, P.R. Woolcock**

*Houghton Poultry Research Station, Huntingdon, Cambridgeshire, PE17 2DA, United Kingdom.
**The Animal Health Trust, Newmarket, Suffolk, CB8 7PN, United Kingdom.

ABSTRACT

Two poorly recognised disease conditions of young Pekin meat ducks are described: the duck fatty kidney syndrome (DFKS) and focal pancreatic necrosis (FPN). The DFKS caused mortalities of up to 30% in individual flocks in Britain between 1978 and 1982. Two distinct age groups were affected but the pathology was similar in both. When 1-day-old ducklings were infected with virulent duck hepatitis virus (DHV) the first birds to die had the liver haemorrhages of classical duck viral hepatitis (DVH). In contrast the last birds to die had the signs of the DFKS. Some of the birds which survived infection had FPN.

A virus was isolated from the pancreas of a bird taken from a DFKS outbreak. The virus caused FPN in ducklings after triple plaque purification in duck embryo kidney cells. It was shown to be an enterovirus which cross-neutralised with DHV type I. Another virus was isolated from ducklings on a farm where DVH had not been recorded and where DHV vaccine had not been used. The virus caused lethal DVH and DFKS when inoculated into 1-day-old ducklings, together with FPN in the survivors. The occurrence of virulent DHV on a farm without hepatitis is discussed.

INTRODUCTION.

In 1978 mortalities of up to 30% occurred in flocks of Pekin meat ducklings in the United Kingdom. Birds in the affected flocks were vaccinated as 1-day-olds with the H55 duck hepatitis virus (DHV) vaccine (Crighton and Woolcock, 1978) and classical duck viral hepatitis (DVH) was not seen in the birds. Affected birds became listless and stopped eating. Within 1 hour they were in sternal recumbancy and occasionally showed extreme opisthotonus. Once a bird became ill it died very rapidly. All the mortalities in the 1 to 2 week age group occurred within a 3 day period but in the 5 to 6 week age group the mortalities could be spread over 7 to 10 days. The surviving birds grew on to be a flock of uniform-sized birds. Histologically the dead birds had esterified lipid basal to the nuclei of the renal proximal tubules and in the macrophages of the splenic white pulp. These findings suggested a severe lipaemia of limited duration. The

†This work was funded by a grant from the Duck Producers Association through the British Poultry Federation. The research was conducted at The Animal Health Trust, Newmarket, Suffolk, United Kingdom.

livers of the dead birds occasionally showed focal necrotising hepatitis with little inflammatory reaction. Bile duct hyperplasia was common in the survivors. Kapp, Karsai and Weiner (1969) reported fat in the kidneys of birds infected with DHV so it was decided to investigate DHV as a possible cause of the duck fatty kidney syndrome (DFKS), regardless of the vaccination status of the birds.

During that study focal pancreatic necrosis (FPN) was occasionally seen as an incidental finding in birds which survived infection with DHV. Strelnikov (1970) described necrotic lesions in the pancreas of birds infected with DHV suggesting an association between DVH and FPN. However, when FPN was seen on a farm where hepatitis did not occur it was decided to isolate the causative virus and examine its relationship to classical DHV type I.

MATERIALS AND METHODS.

Birds

1-day-old ducklings from parents without antibodies to DHV were purchased from a commercial source. They were housed on wood shavings in metal-sided floor pens with all the groups in one room, including the controls. The hyperimmune chicken serum was raised against triple plaque purified viruses in SPF Rhode Island Red chicks from Houghton Poultry Research Station, Cambridgeshire.

Virology

The virulent Q strain of DHV was isolated in England in 1964 (Asplin, 1965a) and stored as an infected liver homogenate at $-70^{\circ}C$. The H55 vaccine was commercial vaccine. The PB virus was isolated in duck embryo kidney (DEK) cells from the pancreas of a 7-day-old duckling during a DFKS outbreak. The bird had been vaccinated with H55 at 1-day-old. The PD virus was isolated in DEK cells from a pool of the pancreases of four 4-week-old ducklings which had not been vaccinated. The DEK cell cultures were produced by the method of Woolcock, Chalmers and Davis (1982).

Farms

Farm B had well maintained, controlled environment poultry houses in which either broiler chickens or ducklings were raised. Geese were also raised intensively in some houses from May to December. Additional ducks and geese were occasionally raised in open fields. Ducklings were purchased from two sources, sometimes simultaneously but usually separately. British ducklings were from parents without antibodies to DHV and were vaccinated with the H55 vaccine on arrival. Danish ducklings possessed maternal immunity to DHV and were not vaccinated on the farm.

Farm D was a multi-age site with breeding ducks and the offspring in close proximity. The adults had contact with wild birds. Ducklings were initially raised in wooden sheds but from 4 weeks of age they were transferred to houses with wire meshed sides. The birds were not vaccinated against DHV.

Experimental Design

In the DFKS pathogenesis experiment 100 1-day-old ducklings were given one LD50 of the virulent Q strain of DHV subcutaneously. Ten live birds were selected at 6, 24, 48, 72 and 120 hours post-infection and any dead birds were collected at those times. Twenty-two control birds were not infected and were collected at appropriate times. Oil red O stains were made of frozen sections of liver, spleen and kidney from each bird, and Nile blue sulphate stains were made to determine whether the fat was esterified.

RESULTS

Of the 100 ducklings given one LD50 of Q virus, 47 died within 72 hours of infection. Liver haemorrhages were the only presenting post-mortem signs in 25 birds, 24 of which died before 48 hours. From 48-72 hours grossly distended pale kidneys were present in 20 birds, 14 of which also had liver haemorrhages. The other 6 birds which died between 48 and 72 hours had no haemorrhages on the liver but had grossly swollen pale kidneys, the signs of the DFKS (Figure 1). Of the 53 birds killed, only three showed gross lesions, one with liver haemorrhages, one with fatty kidneys and one with FPN. None of the control birds developed gross lesions.

Of the 47 dead birds, 42 had abnormal amounts of fat in the basal region of the renal proximal convoluted tubular epithelial cells (Figure 2). Of the 53 birds killed 13 had fat in the tubular epithelial cells. One control bird had marginal amounts of fat in the renal tubules.

The pancreas from which the PB virus was isolated is shown in Figure 3. The homogenised pancreas was injected subcutaneously into 20 1-day-old ducklings, 5 of which developed FPN by 14 days. Twenty non-injected control birds remained normal. Subsequent duckling passages of affected pancreas homogenates resulted in an increase in the incidence of FPN to 80% in the fourth passage. Five to 7 days after infection numerous round grey to white foci of up to 2mm diameter could be seen throughout the pancreas. Histologically there was a gradual transformation from normal exocrine cells on the edge of a necrotic focus to necrotic cells in the centre (Figure 4). There was very little inflammatory reaction until 7 days after infection when mononuclear cells and fibrosis became apparent. By the seventh passage classical DVH was produced but 6 of the 7 survivors had FPN. At no stage during this study did FPN occur in uninfected control ducklings.

Administration of hyperimmune duck anti-H55 serum subcutaneously 24 hours before or at the time of challenge with an affected pancreas homogenate reduced the number of birds which developed FPN from 11 of 15 birds without serum to 1 of 16 birds with serum. When serum was administered 24 or 48 hours after infection 10 out of 16 birds developed FPN.

Vaccination with H55 vaccine completely protected 10 birds from subsequent challenge when given an affected pancreas homogenate 72 hours after vaccination. Fifteen non-vaccinated birds were challenged at the same time and 10 developed FPN. Ten birds which received vaccine only and 10 which were not infected did not develop FPN.

The PB virus was triple plaque purified and the cloned virus was resistant to treatment with IUDR, chloroform, and pH 3 and had a particle diameter of about 25nm. In cross-neutralisation studies using hyperimmune chicken serum raised against either triple plaque purified PB or H55 viruses, the two cloned viruses could not be distinguished. PB virus was therefore considered to be an enterovirus in the duck hepatitis type I group.

One of the PB virus clones which had been plaque passaged three times in DEK cells caused liver haemorrhages, DFKS and FPN when inoculated into 1-day-old ducklings. In contrast Q virus rapidly lost virulence on plaque passage in DEK cells. The first plaques killed 22 of 35 infected birds (63%), but the second plaques killed only 1 of 47 birds (2%). Subsequent passage in DEK cells resulted in nonlethal plaques.

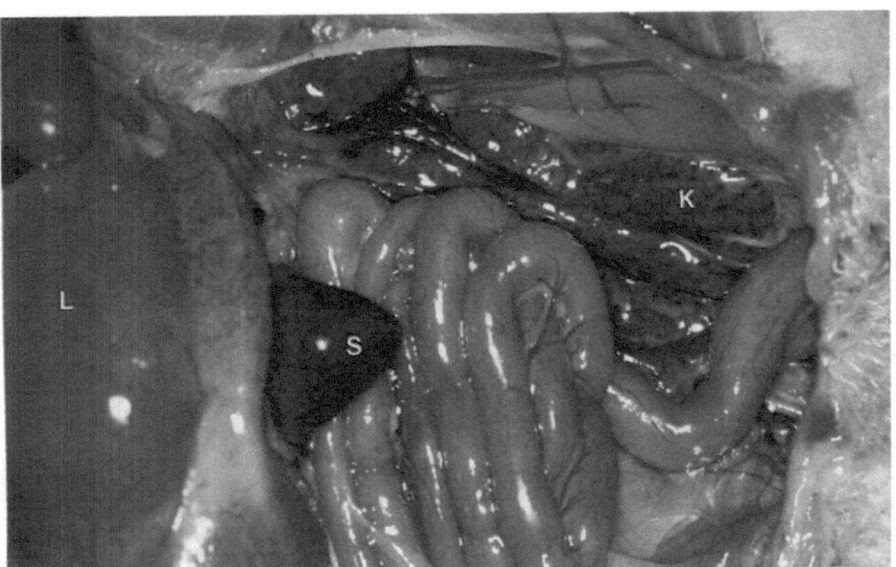

Fig. 1 Typical gross pathology of the DFKS. The liver (L) has no haemorrhages and the spleen (S) is large and mottled. The architecture of the kidneys (K) is accentuated by the pale fat in the tubules. (Photograph courtesy of Avian Pathology.)

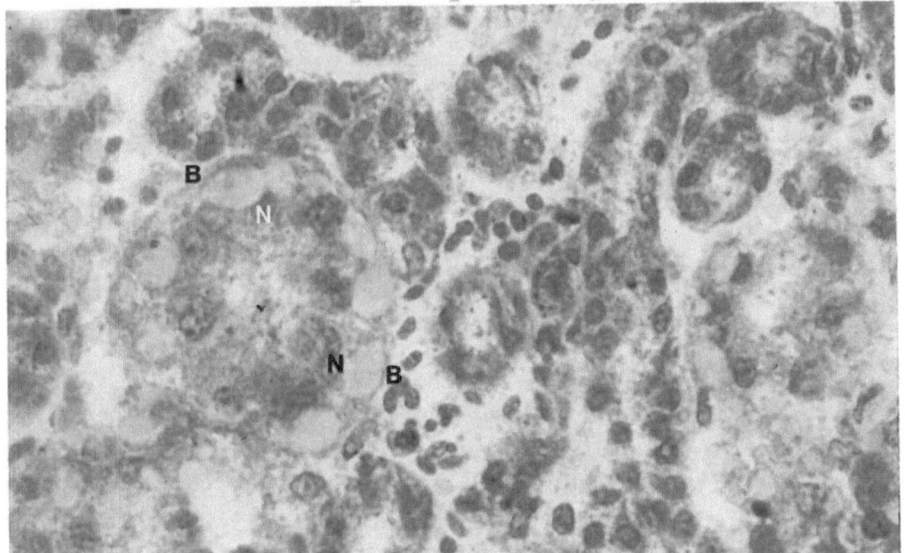

Fig. 2 Frozen section of the kidney from a case of the DFKS stained with Nile blue sulphate. The fat between the nuclei (N) and the basement membrane (B) is stained red indicating esterified fat. Nile blue sulphate x 640.

Cloacal swabs from Farm D, where DVH had never been seen, caused plaques when used to infect DEK cell monolayers. Those plaques caused no lesions when injected subcutaneously into ducklings, but passage of livers from the infected birds resulted in acute DVH and FPN. Passage of control bird livers had no effect. On a subsequent visit to the farm, 6 abnormally small 4-week-old birds were examined and 4 had FPN. The affected pancreases were homogenised and caused plaques on DEK monolayers. Two clones were derived from those plaques, one of which caused FPN in 7 of 10 infected birds. The other clone caused FPN in only 1 of 10. Uninfected control birds showed no changes.

DISCUSSION

The clinical signs and histological changes seen in the DFKS outbreaks were indicative of subacute infections with DHV. However the lack of liver haemorrhages, the vaccination status of the flocks and the fact that 6-week-old birds were dying all indicated non-typical DVH. The virulent Q virus used in this study was collected over two decades before the 1978 DFKS outbreak and was therefore unlikely to be contaminated by a recently evolved strain of antigenically distinct DHV. When Q virus was inoculated into 1-day-old ducklings clinical symptoms and pathological changes similar to those of the DFKS were produced, but in conjunction with the liver haemorrhages typical of DVH. It is possible that the vaccine given to the birds in the field was sufficient to prevent all the aspects of DVH from being expressed so that only the DFKS was seen. If that was the case it should be possible to produce just the DFKS without liver haemorrhage by vaccinating ducklings and challenging them before the protection was complete. That work was not attempted as it is not possible to distinguish between the vaccine and virulent viruses in vitro.

At the time of this study only three duck farms in the United Kingdom were free of DVH. On two of these, their geographical isolation and the stringent disease precautions adopted could be considered to be the reasons for the hepatitis-free status. However the third farm, Farm D, was close to several infected farms and vehicles passed freely between these and Farm D. Farm D was therefore investigated to determine why the disease did not occur. A virus isolated from cloacal swabs from normal birds caused DVH and FPN when passaged in ducklings. Because of the known association between DVH and FPN (Strelnikov, 1970) and the fact that affected pancreases had often lost a considerable amount of the functional exocrine capacity, it seemed reasonable to assume that birds with FPN might grow more slowly than normal. When abnormally small birds were sought a majority had FPN.

Unfortunately the work was terminated at this stage because of lack of funding, but three important questions remained to be answered. Firstly, since DHV is a rapidly spreading virulent virus why is it that birds on Farm D carried this virus in the pancreas but classical virus hepatitis was not seen? Is it possible that a variant field virus existed which was pathogenic enough to be spread and cause FPN but not DVH and that all the new birds became naturally vaccinated on arrival? Farm D was a multiage site so such an agent could be maintained in the duckling population.

The second question is, if the DFKS is a subacute form of DVH why did it appear in vaccinated birds? The vaccine was made from the same seed virus before, during and after the outbreak so it is unlikely to have been contaminated. The incidence of the syndrome decreased in 1982, and in 1983 DHV type II, an astro-like virus which is antigenically distinct from the DHV type I enterovirus, was isolated (Gough et al., 1984). Both viruses caused similar disease symptoms (Gough et al., 1985) so it is conceivable that the 1978 outbreak of the DFKS could have been due to DHV type II.

Several British farms were purchasing 1-day-old ducklings with maternal immunity to DHV type I from abroad at the time of the DFKS outbreak. It is interesting to note that the only other time DVH type II has been a problem was in 1964 (Asplin, 1965b) shortly after the introduction of maternal vaccination in the UK (Asplin, 1956). From 1965 onwards most farms bought type I susceptible ducklings and vaccinated them on arrival with a live attenuated type I vaccine. However, those farms with disease problems often imported maternally immune birds. Could it be that the live type I vaccine had a competitive inhibition effect against DHV type II and that is why DHV type II remained dormant for the two decades in which the live vaccine was used?

The third question is why subacute DVH occurred in 5 to 6-week-old birds when age immunity to DHV usually begins at 4 weeks (Asplin, 1956)? Birds in this older group usually had conjunctivitis associated with Chlamydia psittaci infection (Farmer, Chalmers and Woolcock, 1982) (Figure 5). It is conceivable that a combination of C. psittaci and DHV infection reduced the age immunity to the point where both hepatitis and chlamydiosis

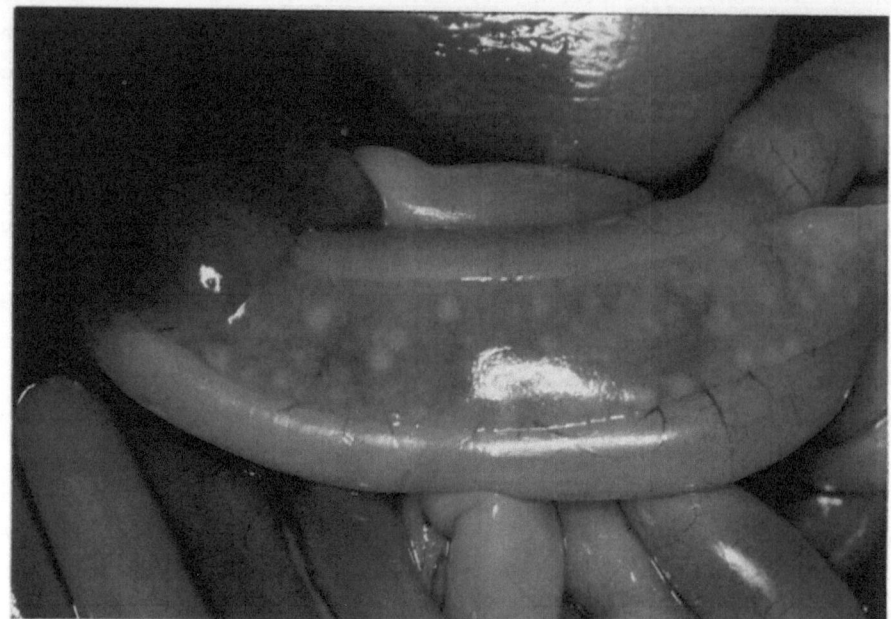

Fig. 3 Focal pancreatic necrosis. The pancreas contains many
grey to white foci of variable sizes up to 2 mm in diameter. The
liver is normal for a 7-day-old duck. (Photograph courtesy of
Avian Pathology.)

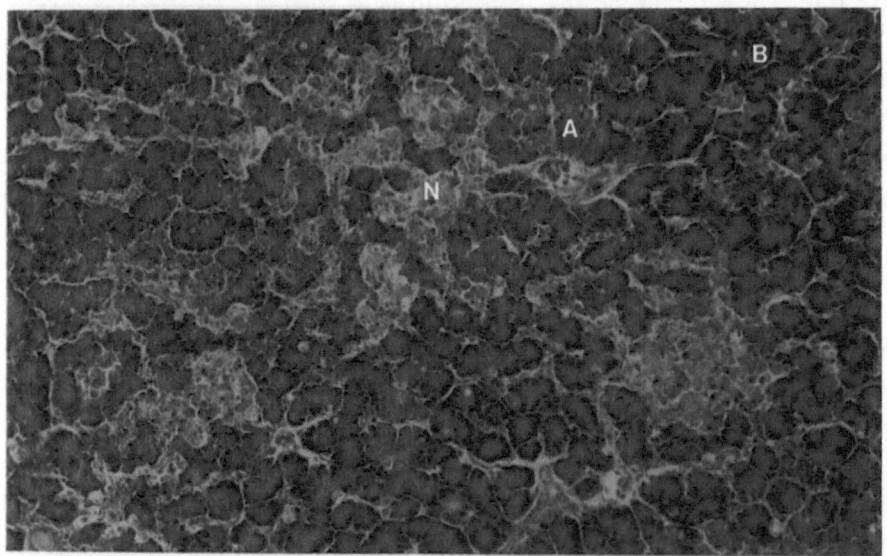

Fig. 4 Focal pancreatic necrosis, 7 days post-infection with
cloned PB virus. There is a transition from normal bicolour
cells (B) through acidophilic cells (A) to a focus of necrosis
(N). H & E x 128. (Photograph courtesy of Avian Pathology.)

221

combined to cause mortalities (Chalmers, Farmer and Woolcock, 1985).

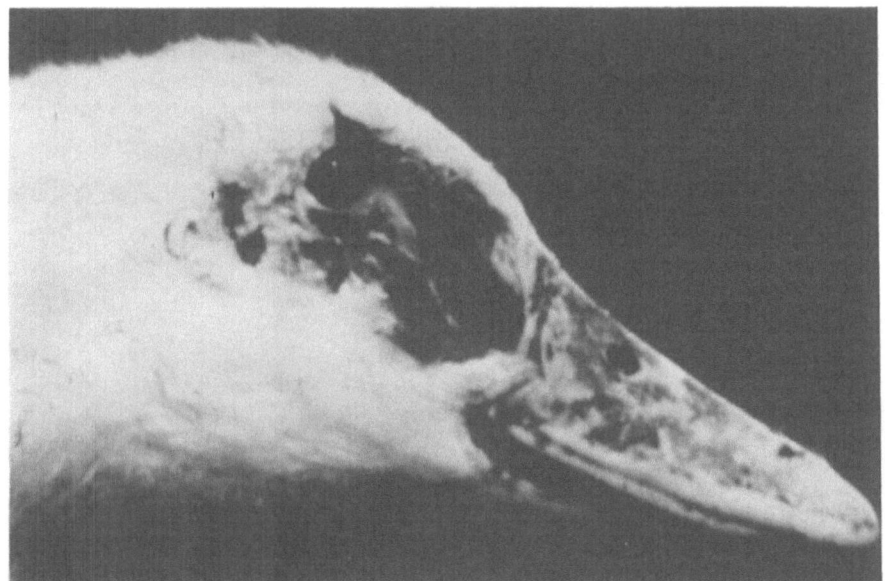

Fig. 5   Conjunctivitis in a 5-week-old duck during a DFKS/FPN outbreak. Chlamydia psittaci was isolated from a conjunctival swab of this bird.

All three questions are of major importance to the duck producers of many countries in the EEC, but further research will be necessary before the answers become available.

BIBLIOGRAPHY

Asplin, F.D. 1956. The production of ducklings resistant to viral hepatitis. Veterinary Record, 68, 412-413.

Asplin, F.D. 1965a. Duck hepatitis. Veterinary Record, 77, 487-488.

Asplin, F.D. 1965b. Duck hepatitis: Vaccination against two serological types. Veterinary Record, 77, 1529-1530.

Chalmers, W.S.K., Farmer, H. and Woolcock, P.R. 1985. Duck hepatitis virus and Chlamydia psittaci outbreak. Veterinary Record, 116, 223.

Crighton, G.W. and Woolcock, P.R. 1978. Active immunisation of ducklings against duck virus hepatitis. Veterinary Record, 102, 358-361.

Farmer, H., Chalmers, W.S.K. and Woolcock, P.R. 1982. Chlamydia psittaci isolated from the eyes of domestic ducks (Anas platyrhynchos) with conjunctivitis and rhinitis. Veterinary Record, 110, 59.

Gough, R.E., Collins, M.S., Borland, E.D. and Keymer, I.F. 1984. Astrovirus-like particles associated with hepatitis in ducklings. Veterinary Record, 114, 279.

Gough, R.E., Borland, E.D., Keymer, I.F. and Stuart, J.S. 1985. An outbreak of Duck Hepatitis type II in Commercial ducks. Avian Pathology, 14, 227-236.

Kapp, P., Karsai, F. and Weiner, I. 1969. On the pathogenesis of duckling hepatitis. Acta Veterinaria Academiae Scientiarum Hungericae, 19, 217-227.

Strelnikov, A.P. 1970. Pathological changes in the pancreas of ducks with viral hepatitis. Trudy Moskovskoi Veterinarnoi Akademii, 54, 69-70.

Woolcock, P.R., Chalmers, W.S.K. and Davis, D. 1982. A plaque assay for duck hepatitis virus. Avian Pathology, 11, 607-610.

DUCK HEPATITIS TYPE 2 ASSOCIATED WITH AN ASTROVIRUS

R.E. Gough.
Central Veterinary Laboratory
New Haw, Weybridge, Surrey
KT15 3NB England

ABSTRACT

A disease of ducks, characterised by hepatitis, caused losses of up to 50% in 6 to 14 day-old-ducks and up to 25% in 4 to 6-week old ducks. During the period under investigation total losses exceeded 40,000 ducks. The affected ducks were the offspring of parents that had received duck hepatitis type 1 vaccine.

Examination of livers and faeces from infected ducks by electron microscopy resulted in the detection of numerous astrovirus-like particles. Repeated passage in the amniotic sac of embryonating specific-pathogen-free chicken eggs resulted in the isolation and detection of the astrovirus in the embryo livers.

The results of cross protection and challenge tests indicate that the astrovirus and duck hepatitis type 2 virus are antigenically similar. Laboratory investigations with an attenuated chicken embryo adapted duck hepatitis type 2 vaccine have shown that the vaccine confers protection against challenge with the duck astrovirus.

It is suggested that the disease known as duck hepatitis type 2 is caused by an astrovirus and hereafter should be referred to as duck astrovirus infection.

INTRODUCTION

A disease caused by an agent serologically distinct from classical duck virus hepatitis (DVH) was widespread in 2 to 6-week-old ducks on fattening fields in East Anglia, England from 1963 to 1968 (Mansi *et al*, 1964; Asplin, 1965a). To differentiate the two diseases it was suggested by Asplin (1965b) that the virus causing classical DVH be referred to as duck hepatitis (DH) type I virus and the new serotype as duck hepatitis (DH) type 2 virus.

By 1969 DH type 2 was no longer reported to occur in England. However, during 1983 a serious disease occurred on a duck farm in East Anglia resulting in losses of between 10 and 25% in 4 to 6-week-old ducks and up to 50% in 6 to 14-day-old ducks.

This report describes the clinical and virological findings following investigation of the disease.

MATERIALS AND METHODS

Stock

The farm received day-old ducklings weekly that were the offspring of parents that had received DH type 1 vaccine. The ducks were
reared inside until 3 to 4 weeks old and then fattened on fields until
slaughter. During the winter the ducks were reared entirely inside.

Virological examination

Twenty per cent (w/v) suspensions of selected organs were prepared
and inoculated into embryonating chicken and duck eggs, also confluent
monolayers of duck kidney and chicken embryo liver tissue cultures, as
described (Gough et al, 1985). Livers and faeces from dead ducks were
prepared and examined by direct electron microscopy (Gough et al,
1985).

Serological tests

Several samples from ducks that had survived the disease were sero
tested for the presence of DH Type 1 (Gough and Spackman, 1981) and DH
type 2 neutralising antibodies (Gough et al, 1985)

Transmission studies

Twenty per cent (w/v) suspensions of infected livers were prepared
in antibiotic saline and inoculated subcutaneously into 20, 2 to 3-day-
old susceptible ducklings. No bacterial growth was detected in the
inoculum.

Cross protection studies

The relationship between DH type 1, DH type 2 and the duck astrovirus was studied by cross protection and challenge tests in ducklings
using DH type 1 and 2 vaccines and reference challenge viruses. The
details have been published elsewhere (Gough et al, 1985).

RESULTS

Clinical history and postmortem findings

The problem started in 4 to 6-week-old ducks in rearing fields on
a farm in Norfolk, with losses of between 10 and 25%. Subsequently 6
to 14-day-old ducks reared inside became affected with losses of up to

50%. Ducklings died within 1 to 2 hours of appearing sick, showing acute opisthotonos. Many of the birds exhibited polydypsia and droppings were often loose and white. Survivors reared normally.

Postmortem and histopathological findings have been reported in detail elsewhere (Gough *et al*, 1985). Briefly, both macroscopically and histologically the disease had similarities with DH Type 1. Multiple haemorrhages in the livers were common, some were punctate and others formed confluent bands across the surface of the organ. The kidneys were often swollen, with the blood vessels injected and standing out from the pale kidney substance.

Histologically there was a widespread necrosis of the hepatocyte cytoplasm with bile duct hyperplasia present in varying degrees.

Virological results

Electron microscopy examination of liver and faeces from dead ducks revealed large aggregates of round virus particles 28-30 nm in diameter. The largest aggregates were seen in the liver preparations (Fig 1). On the basis of size and morphology the particles resembled astroviruses (Gough *et al*, 1984).

After 4 passages of the original liver suspensions in the amniotic-sac of embryonating SPF chicken eggs a number of the embryos appeared inert and stunted, six to 10 days after inoculation. Many of the stunted embryos had green necrotic livers. Examination of suspensions of infected embryo livers by electron microscopy revealed astrovirus-like particles. No viruses were isolated from livers and kidney suspension following repeated passage in duck kidney amd chicken embryo liver tissue cultures.

Using a suspension of concentrated infected embryo livers in amnio-allantoic fluid a virus neutralisation test was performed in embryonating SPF chicken eggs against DH type I antiserum. No reduction in infectivity was recorded.

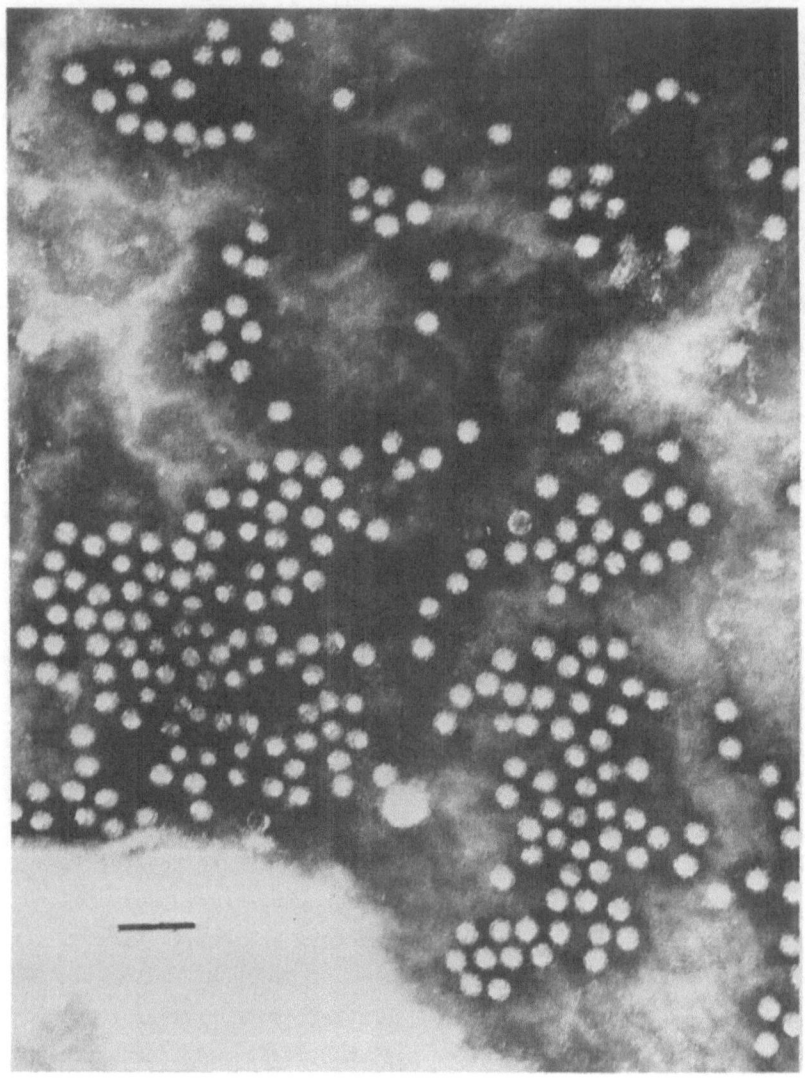

Fig 1. Astrovirus-like particles in liver suspension from ducklings with hepatitis. Bar represents 100nm.

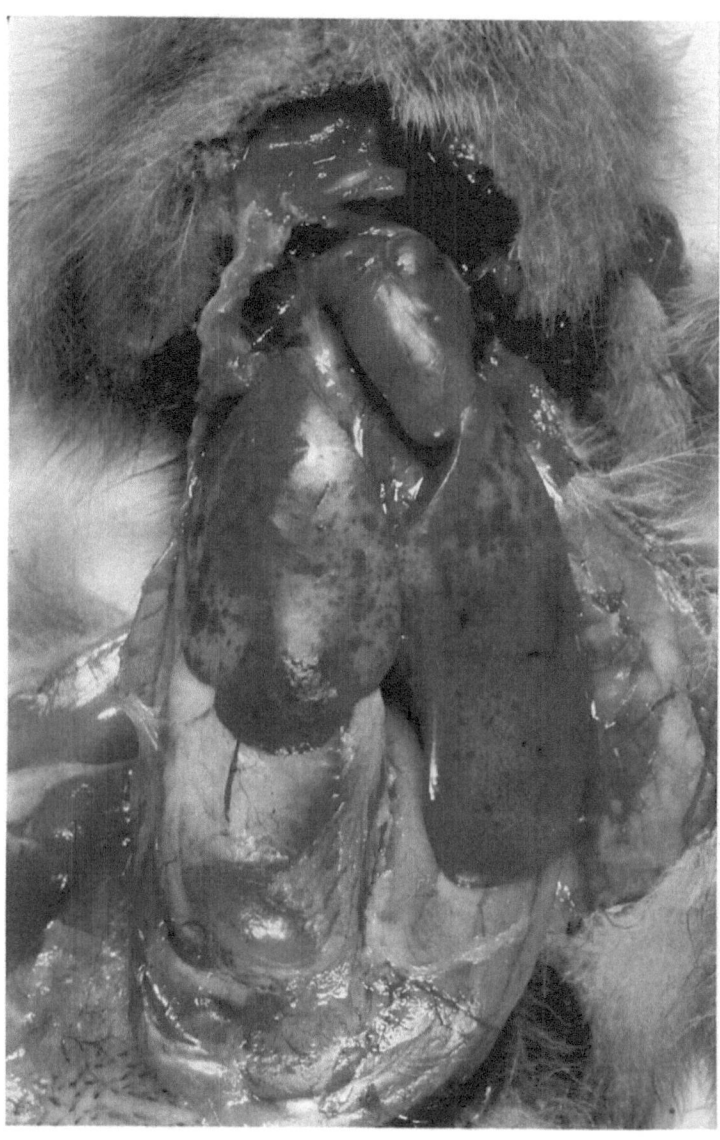

Fig 2. Liver lesions in 10-day old duckling that had died from duck hepatitis type II infection.

Serology

No neutralising antibodies to DH type 1 virus were detected in serum samples from ducks that had survived the disease. However, low levels of antibody to DH type 2 virus were detected.

Transmission study results

Of the 20 ducklings infected experimentally, five died between 2 and 4 days after incoluation showing gross and microscopic lesions in the liver and kidneys similar to those seen in field cases. Electron microscope examination of suspensions of affected livers revealed numerous astrovirus-like particles. Some aggregates contained more than 10^3 virus particles. No virus particles were detected in livers from normal, age-matched controls. Serial passage of the astrovirus in ducklings resulted in mortality levels ranging from 25 to 55%.

Cross protection results

The results of cross protection studies are presented in Table 1. The results show that DH type 2 and the duck astrovirus are antigenically similar but both are unrelated to duck DH type 1.

TABLE 1   Results of cross protection studies with duck hepatitis (DH) type 1 and 2, and the duck astrovirus isolate

Vaccines	Challenge Viruses		
	DH type I (Asplin, 1958)	DH type 2 (Asplin, 1965b)	Duck astrovirus (Gough, 1984)
DH type 1 (Crighton & Woolcock, 1978)	0/20 [a]	3/20	4/20
DH type 2 (Asplin, 1965b)	11/19	0/20	0/20
None	6/10	5/17	10/35

a - Number died over number in group.

DISCUSSION

From the results of this investigation it is concluded that the serious disease of ducks reported here was duck hepatitis type 2. The disease was last observed in 1969 (Asplin, unpublished) and there have been no published reports of the disease occurring since then. The absence of the disease during the intervening period is not fully understood. In the outbreak reported here the ducks reared on fields were the first to die of the disease, suggesting contact with wild birds, particularly species of corvidae and seagulls, as a possible source of infection. The absence of the disease during the winter months, when the ducks are reared inside, further strengthens this view. Further outbreaks of the disease have been confirmed on two other duck fattening farms in East Anglia, affecting 3 to 6-week-old ducks reared in fields.

The presence of astrovirus-like particles in the livers of affected ducklings is of interest. Similar viruses have been detected by electron microscopy in the faeces of a number of mammalian species and turkey poults (McNulty *et al*, 1980). However, the detection and cultivation of astroviruses from ducklings with hepatitis is thought to be an original observation.

Astroviruses have also been detected by electron microscopy in material derived from the original DH type 2 isolates, described by Asplin (1965b). It is concluded therefore that the etiological agent of DH type 2 infection is an astrovirus, and the name duck astrovirus is suggested to differentiate the disease from duck virus hepatitis.

Further studies are in progress to characterise the duck astrovirus using physical and biochemical tests, and to compared it with astroviruses from other species.

REFERENCES

Asplin, F.D. (1958). An attenuated strain of duck hepatitis virus. Vet. Record., 70, 1226-1230.
Asplin, F.D. (1965a). Duck hepatitis. Vet. Record., 77, 487-488.
Asplin, F.D. (1965b). Duck hepatitis : Vaccination against two serological types. Vet. Record., 77, 1529-1530.
Crighton, G.W. and Woolcock, P.R. (1978). Active immunisation of ducklings against duck virus hepatitis. Vet. Record., 102, 358-361.

Gough, R.E. and Spackman, D. (1981). Studies with inactivated duck
   virus hepatitis vaccines in breeder ducks. Avian Path.,
   10, 477-479.
Gough, R.E., Collins, M.S., Borland, E.D. and Keymer, I.F. (1984).
   Astrovirus-like particles associated with hepatitis in ducklings.
   Vet. Rec., 144, 279.
Gough, R.E., Borland, E.D., Keymer, I.F. and Stuart, J.C. (1985). An
   outbreak of duck hepatitis type 2 in commercial ducks. Avian
   Path., 14, 227-236.
Mansi, W., Schofield, P.B. and Gonzalez, V.C. (1964). Duckling virus
   infection. Vet. Record., 76, 740.
McNulty, M.S., Curran, W.L. and McFerran, J.B. (1980). Detection of
   astroviruses in turkey faeces by direct electron microscopy.
   Vet. Record., 106, 561.

DUAL INFECTIONS OF DUCKS WITH DERZSY'S DISEASE
AND EDS (A-127) VIRUSES

A. Cakala*, F. Coudert**, E. Salamanowicz*, L. Cauchy**

*Institytut Weterynarii, 57 Al.partyzantow, Pulawy, Pologne.
** I.N.R.A. Station de Pathologie aviaire et de Parasitologie,
37380 Monnaie, France.

ABSTRACT

Muscowy ducklings were infected with a very pathogenic parvovirus, Derzsy's Disease Virus (DDV) and an adenovirus of a type frequently isolated from ducks (EDS 76) - (A-127). 3 groups of ducklings were respectively infected with DDV plus A-127, DDV, A-127, and a control group was raised under similar conditions. Pathological signs were observed and body weights recorded. Sera were collected weekly and analyzed for DDV and A-127 antibodies. In addition, in vitro assays of multiplication of these viruses on duck embryo fibroblasts were conducted. In ducklings, dual infection increases the mortality rate and depresses the body weight gain, as compared to infection with either virus alone. The humoral response did not appear to be influenced by dual infection. No difference in cytopathogenic effects were detected in vitro between single and dual infections.

INTRODUCTION

Mixed viral infections appear frequently in birds. The most severe disease entity in growing Moscowy ducklings and goslings is Derzsy's disease caused by a parvovirus. Adenoviruses were also isolated from geese (Kisary, 1974; Zsak et al., 1984), ducks (Bartha, 1984; McFerran et al., 1977a; McFerran et al., 1977b) and Muscowy ducks (Bouquet et al., 1982; Malkinson et al., 1980). The results of a serological survey carried out in France by Marius et al. (1983) have shown that 50% of examined Moscowy ducks had high antibody levels to the egg drop syndrome 1976 adenovirus (A-127).

The aim of this experiment was to investigate the effect of infection with strain A-127 and a virulent strain of Parvovirus in Muscowy ducklings. The interaction between these two viruses was also investigated in vitro.

MATERIALS AND METHODS

Birds

Ninety-five one-day-old Muscowy ducklings derived from an SPF duck flock were used. This flock was maintained in isolated housing with a positive pressure ventilation system.

Virus strains

A virulent strain of Derzsy's disease virus (DDV) was obtained from Dr Marius (Laboratoire de Pathologie aviaire, Ploufragan, France). The LD_{50} of this strain for goslings was $10^{6.5}$.

Strain B-38 of DDV adapted to goose embryo fibroblasts was kindly supplied by Dr Kisary (Academy of Sciences, Budapest, Hungary). This strain was passaged three times in Muscowy duck embryo fibroblasts (MDEF) and its $TCID_{50}$ was $10^{5.0}$ in 0.1 ml.

Strain A-127 of avian adenovirus was received from Dr Vielitz (Lohmann, Cuxhaven, West Germany). This strain was adapted to chick embryo kidney cell culture and passaged 5 times in MDEF culture; its HA titre was $\log_2 4$.

The same strain, before using for infection of ducklings, was propagated in duckling embryo liver cells; $TCID_{50}$ of this strain was $10^{5.0}$ in 0.1 ml.

Muscowy duck embryo fibroblasts culture (MDEF)

The cultures were prepared from 17-day-old embryos. The cells were grown in a mixture of MEM medium with 10 per cent calf serum and 1 per cent bacto-tryptose-phosphate (BTP).

Determination of virus titres

$TCID_{50}$ of Derzsy's disease virus: Tenfold dilutions of virus in maintenance medium were made. Each dilution was pipetted into five replicate wells of microculture plates. MDEF suspension was added to each well. Plates were placed in a humidified incubator with 5 per cent CO_2 at 37°C. Cell monolayers were examined with an inverted microscope to detect cytopathic effect (CPE). Virus titre was calculated according to the Reed-Muench method. HA titre of A-127 strain: the test was performed according to McFerran et al. (1978), using 1 per cent suspension of chicken erythrocytes in PBS and twofold dilutions of virus materials (microtitre system).

Serological tests

Haemagglutination inhibition test (HI) was performed according to McFerran et al. (1978) using 1 per cent chicken red blood cells, double dilutions of serum (initial dilution 1:2) and 4 HA-units of the virus. All sera titres higher than 2^3 were considered as positive.

Virus neutralisation tests (VN) were carried out as described by Marius et al. (1983) and Kisary (1974). Twofold serial dilutions of sera diluted 1:10 were mixed with equal volumes of 100 $TCID_{50}$ of virus and incubated at 37°C for 1h. Five wells of microculture plates per dilution were inoculated with serum-virus mixture. Cell cultures infected only with virus or serum served as controls. The highest dilution of serum neutralising 50 per cent of virus was considered SND_{50}.

All experiments in vitro were repeated 3 times and the results were expressed as mean geometrical values.

RESULTS

Experiment in vivo

Effect of A-127 adenovirus infection in Muscowy ducklings infected with Derzsy's disease virus (DDV).

One-day-old ducklings were divided into the following groups: group I - 39-day-old ducklings were inoculated orally and intratracheally with A-127 virus dose 10^5 $TCID_{50}$ per bird, and then at 10 days old infected i.m. with 0.5 ml of DDV ($10^{6.5}$ LD_{50} diluted 1.300000), group II - 30 ducklings, 10-day-old infected i.m. with the same dose of DDV, group III - 13 ducklings infected on the first day of life with A-127 virus. group IV - 13 uninfected ducklings.

All birds were observed for 6 weeks. The clinical symptoms and mortality due to Derzsy's disease virus were observed in ducklings of group I and group II. In group II infected only with DDV,12 ducklings died whereas in group I - infected with DDV and A-127,18 ducklings died (table 1).

After 6 weeks all ducklings were weighed and the mean weight gains in each group were calculated (table 2). The mean weight of uninfected ducklings was 1752 g whereas the mean weight of ducklings in the group dually infected with A-127 and DDV was 894 g. The difference between these two groups was 858 g. The ducklings inoculated only with DDV weighed 1074 g. This differs from the mean weight of ducklings with the dual infection by about 180 g.

TABLE 1   Losses among ducklings infected with EDS-76 and Derzsy's
disease (DDV) viruses.

Virus – age of infection	Number of ducklings	Mortality						Total	%
		1^x	2	3	4	5	6		
EDS-1 day)) 39 DDV-10 days)	39	1	2	2	2	5	6	18	46,15
DDV-10 days	30	–	–	7	2	2	1	12	40,0
EDS-1 day	13	–	1	–	–	–	–	1	7,14
Uninfected	13	–	–	–	–	–	–	–	0

x – weeks of age

TABLE 2   The mean weight of ducklings infected with A-127 and
Derzsy's disease (DDV) viruses.

Virus – age of infection	Mean weight at 6 weeks of age in g
A-127 1 day DDV 10 days	894
DDV 10 days	1074
A-127 1 day	1750
Uninfected	1752

At weekly intervals the sera from ducklings of each group were collected and the VN test with DDV and HI test with A-127 virus were conducted.
The results of serological investigations are summarized in figs. 1 and
2. Serological responses to DDV in ducklings inoculated with DDV only or
dually with A-127 virus did not differ significantly. The highest SND_{50}
mean titre in group I was found 32 days p.i. On the other hand in group
II, ducklings inoculated only with DDV, the highest SND_{50} titre was shown
25 days p.i. The highest serum titre in ducklings of both groups was
$2^{11.3}$.

The HI antibody titres against A-127 virus were not high. The positive titres, above $log_2 3$ were noted earlier, just 7 days p.i., in the sera
of ducklings infected only with A-127 strain, whereas in the group of
ducklings with dual infection the first positive reactions were shown in

the second week p.i. The highest HI antibody titre was 2^7 and it was noted
in the 3rd week p.i. in the group with dual infection. In ducklings inoculated only with A-127 the peak titre was noted 2 weeks after infection.
After 3 weeks HI antibodies decreased rapidly and up to 6 weeks remained
at very low levels, ranging from 0 to 2^4.

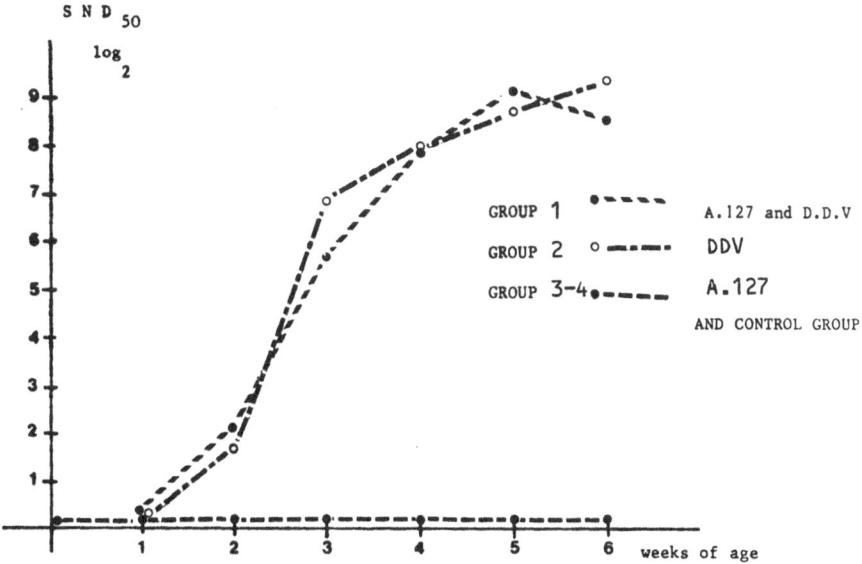

Fig 1. Serological responses to Derzsy's disease virus in inoculated
and control ducklings.

The stated differences in mortality and depressed weight in ducklings
inoculated with the two viruses induced us to carry out an additional in
vitro experiment.

The aim of this experiment was investigate if there was an interaction
between Derzsy's disease virus and A-127 adenovirus in Muscowy duck embryo
fibroblasts culture (MDEF).

In the first trial the MDEF cultures were inoculated simultaneously
with $10^{2.83}$ TCID of DDV strain B-38 and with various doses of A-127 strain
(from $10^{1.3}$ to $10^{5.3}$ $TCID_{50}$).

In the second trial the MDEF cultures were inoculated with $10^{2.83}$
$TCID_{50}$ of DDV and after 24 hours they were infected with several doses of

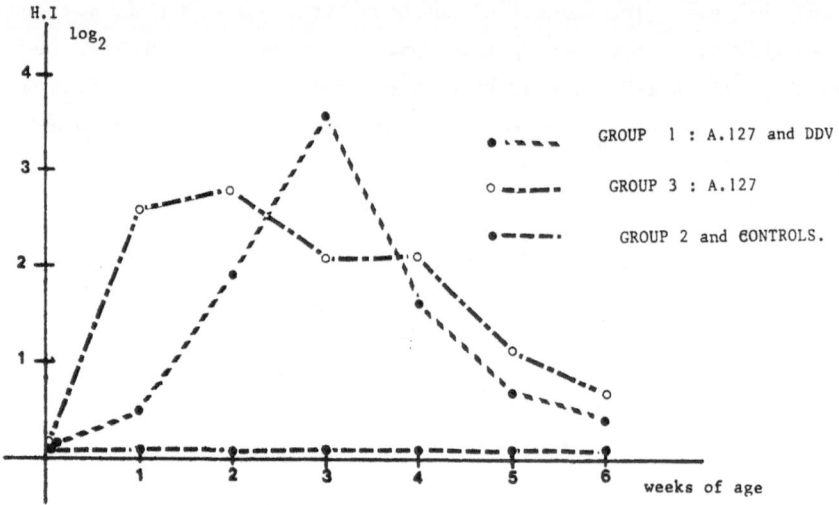

Fig 2.   Serological responses to A-127 adenovirus in inoculated and con-
          trol ducklings.

adenovirus ranging from $10^{1.3}$ to $10^{5.3}$ $TCID_{50}$.

In the third trial the MDEF cultures were inoculated with several doses
ranging from $10^{1.3}$ to $10^{5.3}$ $TCID_{50}$ of A-127 strain and after 24 hours they
were infected with DDV in a dose of $10^{2.83}$ $TCID_{50}$. As controls, the MDEF
cultures inoculated only with $10^{2.83}$ $TCID_{50}$ of DDV or only with A-127 strain
in several doses, as above were used.

All inoculated cultures were incubated 7 days in a humidified incubator
with 5 per cent CO_2 at 37°C. After 7 days the virus materials of each trial
were collected and the determination of $TCID_{50}$ for DDV or HA titre for
A-127 were conducted.

The results were summarized in tables 3, 4 and 5. No significant
differences in $TCID_{50}$ of DDV propagated in MDEF cultures in the absence or
presence of A-127 virus were shown. Also no differences were found in CPE
in cells when they were infected either with DDV only or with DDV and A-127
strain. Independently of inoculation time of MDEF with A-127 virus simultaneously, prior or after infection with DDV the differences between
$TCID_{50}$ of DDV have not exceeded 0.2 - 0.3 log. Also the dose of inoculated
A-127 virus had no influence on $TCID_{50}$ of DDV.

DISCUSSION

The results of presented experiments indicate that dual infection of Muscowy ducklings caused by adenovirus strain A-127 and pathogenic DDV may exert some influence on the higher mortality rate and the lowered weight gain of these birds. However, in vitro the interaction between these two investigated viruses could not be confirmed.

TABLE 3 Propagation of DDV in the presence of A-127 virus in MDEF cultures (simultaneous infection with DDV and A-127 virus).

Dose of DDV log TCID$_{50}$	Dose of A-127 log TCID$_{50}$	Mean TCID$_{50}$ of DDV		Mean HA titre of A-127	
		with A-127	without A-127	with DDV	without DDV
	5.3	4.5^x	4.7	4^{xx}	4
	4.3	4.7	4.7	4	3
	3.3	4.5	4.5	3	4
2.83	2.3	4.7	4.7	3	3
	1.3	4.3	4.5	2	3
	–	–	5.0	–	–

x - $\log_{10}$

xx - $\log_2$

TABLE 4 Propagation of DDV in the presence of A-127 virus in MDEF cultures (inoculation DDV prior to A-127 virus infection).

Dose of DDV log TCID$_{50}$	Dose of A-127 log TCID$_{50}$	Mean TCID$_{50}$ of DDV		Mean HA titre of A-127	
		with A-127	without A-127	with DDV	without DDV
	5.3	4.5^x	4.5	4^{xx}	4
	4.3	4.2	4.5	3	4
	3.3	4.5	4.7	4	2
2.83	2.3	4.5	4.9	2	3
	1.3	4.7	4.9	2	2
	–	–	4.9	–	–

x - $\log_{10}$

xx - $\log_2$

TABLE 5   Progagation of DDV in the presence of A-127 virus in MDEF
cultures (inoculation of A-127 virus prior to DDV infection).

Dose of DDV log $TCID_{50}$	Dose of A-127 log $TCID_{50}$	Mean $TCID_{50}$ of DDV with A-127	Mean $TCID_{50}$ of DDV without A-127	Mean HA titre of A-127 with DDV	Mean HA titre of A-127 with DDV
	5.3	4.5^x	4.5	4^{xx}	4
	4.3	4.7	4.7	3	4
2.83	3.3	4.7	5.0	3	3
	2.3	4.5	4.8	2	2
	1.3	4.7	4.7	1	1
	–	–	5.0	–	–

x - $\log_{10}$
xx - $\log_2$

ACKNOWLEDGEMENTS

We are greatly indebted to Drs V.Marius, J. Kisary and E. Vielitz for
providing us with the virus strains used in this study.

REFERENCES

Bartha, A. 1984. Dropped egg production in ducks associated with adeno-
     virus infection. Avian Pathol., 13, 119-126.
Bouquet, J.F., Moreau Y., McFerran, J.B. and Connor, T.J. 1982. Isolation
     and characterisation of an adenovirus isolated from Muscowy ducks.
     Avian Pathol., 11, 301-307.
Kisary, J. 1974. Cross neutralization tests on Parvovirus isolated from
     goslings. Avian Pathol., 3, 293-296.
Malkinson, M. and Weisman, Y. 1980. Serological survey for the prevalence
     of antibodies to egg drop syndrome 1976 virus in domesticated and wild
     birds in Israel. Avian Pathol., 9, 421-425.
Marius, V., Bonnaud, P., Guittet, M., Trap, D., Gaumont, R. and Bennejean G.
     1983. Résultats d'une enquête sérologique effectuée en France (Vendee)
     chez le canard à rôtir. Avian Pathol., 12, 419-435.
McFerran, J.B. and Adair, B.M. 1977a. Avian adenovirus. Avian Pathol., 6,
     189-217.
McFerran, J.B. and Connor, T.J. 1977b. Further studies on the classific-
     ation of fowl adenoviruses. Avian Dis., 21, 585-595.
McFerran, J.B., McCracken, R.N., McKillop, E.R., McNulty, M.S. and Collins,
     D.S. 1978. Studies on a depressed egg production syndrome in Northern
     Ireland. Avian Pathol. 7, 35-47.
Zsak, L. and Kisary, J. 1984. Characterisation of adenoviruses isolated
     from geese. Avian Pathol., 13, 253-264.

DIAGNOSIS AND CONTROL OF PARVOVIRUS INFECTION
OF GEESE (DERZSY'S DISEASE)

J. Kisary

Universite Libre de Bruxelles, Faculte des Sciences
Laboratoire de Biophysique et Radiobiologie
1640 Rhode-Saint-Genese, Belgium

ABSTRACT

Derzsy's disease of geese and Muscovy ducks is caused by a single antigenic type of parvovirus. Clinical symptoms develop only in birds aged below 1 month, meanwhile, in older birds a latent infection is established. The main pathological alterations develop in the liver and heart muscle. The disease can be diagnosed by virus isolation in primary goose embryo fibroblast cells or by detecting specific antibodies in neutralisation or agargel precipitin tests. The specific control measures include the hyperimmune treatment of day-old birds or vaccination of the parent flocks.

Derzsy's disease of geese is a fatal disease of goslings and Muscovy ducklings aged below 1 month. In older birds a latent infection is established (Derzsy, 1967; anonym, 1974). The aetiological agent is a virus which taxonomically belongs to the Parvovirus genus of PARVOVIRIDAE (Schettler, 1971a; Kisary and Derzsy 1974). From epidemiological point of view it should be stressed that only one antigenic type of the virus has been found up to now (Kisary, 1974) and the virions, as do other parvoviruses, are highly resistant to heat and chemical agents.

The day-old birds can become infected with the virus either by horizontal or by vertical transmission (Derzsy, 1967). Five-seven days after infection the goslings are listless, reluctant to move and remain around the source of heat. The feed and drinking water intake of such goslings decreases, then ceases completely, and their development is arrested. Diarrhoea is a frequent finding. Deaths first occur between the 8th and 10th day of life, the mortality rate reaches its peak around 15 days. By the 3rd to 4th week of life losses due to the parvovirus infection itself are no longer demonstrable. When the susceptibility of goslings is decreased by a certain level of yolk-derived antibodies the main symptoms are retarded growth (uneven flock) and poor feathering (Schettler, 1971b). In this case the losses are in the 3rd and 4th week of life mainly due to secondary bacterial, fungal, mycoplasmal and viral infections. If goslings with high levels of maternal antibodies become infected they will remain symptomless even after a challenge with a high dose of virulent virus under experimental conditions (Kisary et al., 1978).

Post-mortem examination of the dead birds shows liver and heart muscle degeneration frequently accompanied by ascites (Derzsy, 1967; Schettler, 1971a). The pm findings in birds with some protection due to the yolk-derived antibodies vary according to the nature of secondary invaders.

To set up a reliable diagnosis, the results of epidemiological, clinical, post-mortem and virological examinations should be taken into consideration. A suspected case can be confirmed by isolating the virus from the liver or the heart muscle of a dead bird in primary fibroblast cell culture prepared from 12-14 days goose embryo. However, it has to be emphasized that goose parvovirus, like other self-replicating parvoviruses, can replicate only in cells with extensive DNA synthesis (Kisary, 1979). Therefore, the isolation attempts should be carried out by inoculating subconfluent cell cultures maintained with a medium containing at least 5% fetal calf serum. Since the surviving goslings develop antibodies against the parvovirus, it is also advisable to test sera from the question flock when they are 6 weeks old. The presence of antibodies is a definitive proof of parvovirus infection. For this purpose, the virus-neutralisation test (Kisary, 1974) and agar-gel precipitin test (Gough, 1984) can be used. Upon comparison, the first is more sensitive, however, laboursome and depending on the laying season when embryos are available, the latter is considerably less sensitive, but can be performed at any time. As it was mentioned above, the offspring of infected layers are provided with maternal antibodies preventing the development of signs of the disease. To find this type of flock the most useful method is to detect the maternal antibodies in the sera of 1-3-day-old goslings (Kisary et al., 1975). This is especially recommended when flocks have to be tested for import purposes.

The specific control measures are based on the observation that goslings supplied with maternal antibodies by naturally infected layers can be raised up with minimal losses if the keeping conditions are satisfactory (Derzsy, 1967). To provide day-old goslings with sufficient level of protective antibodies there are two possibilities: either treating them with hyperimmune serum at the hatchery (Derzsy et al., 1970) or vaccinating the layers with a living or inactivated virus vaccine (Kisary et al., 1978). The hyperimmune serum is produced in commercial broiler geese by injecting them s.c./virulent virus at age 31 and 45 days, respectively. The serum is collected when the geese are slaughtered at age 58-60 days. When this method is used it has to be emphasized that the treatment (2 ml serum given s.c.

on the neck) should be carried out as early as possible before the potential horizontal infection. Since the half-life of antibodies provided by the
hyperimmune serum in the treated goslings is about 7 days (Kisary, 1977),
it is advisable to repeat it around 10 days of life. This control measure
is recommended when day-old birds of unvaccinated layers are kept in an infected area. Otherwise, the serum-treatment is laboursome, expensive and,
of course, has no effect on the layers which are spreading the virus by the
transovarial route. To overcome the disadvantages of hyperimmune serum treatment of day-old goslings active immunisation of layers and ganders with
an attenuated virus strain has been developed (Kisary et al., 1978). According to the vaccination scheme the parent flock is vaccinated twice in such
a manner that the second vaccination is performed 1 month before the onset
of laying and the interval between the two vaccinations is 2-3 weeks. By u-
sing this vaccination programme specific protection by maternal antibodies
is provided for day-old goslings during the whole laying season. The maternal antibodies circulate in the blood of the young goslings at nearly the
same level for about 18-20 days by which time the immunological responsive-
ness of the goslings has developed (Kisary, 1977). To prevent the activation of the parvovirus infection in the laying flock it should be vaccinated
once at the end of the laying season. The use of an inactivated vaccine is
advisable in a flock where parvovirus infection has not yet been diagnosed.
However, it should be noted that the immunological response induced by an
inactivated vaccine is significantly milder than that elicited by a living
one (Schettler, 1979).

REFERENCES

anonym, 1974. World's Poultry Science Journal, 31, 157.
Derzsy, D. 1967. A viral disease of goslings. I. Epidemiological, clinical,
      pathological and aetiological studies. Acta Vet.Acad.Sci.Hung., 17,
      443-448.
Derzsy, D., Drèn, Cs., Szedő, Mària, Surjàn, J., Toth, B. and Iro, Emma.
      1970. Viral disease of goslings. III. Isolation, properties and anti-
      genic pattern of the virus strains. Acta Vet.Acad.Sci.Hung., 20, 419-
      428.
Gough, R.E. 1984. Application of the agar gel precipitin and virus neutra-
      lisation tests to the serological study of goose parvovirus. Avian
      Pathol., 13, 501-509.
Kisary, J. 1974. Cross-neutralisation tests on parvoviruses isolated from
      goslings. Avian Pathol., 3, 293-296.
Kisary, J. and Derzsy, D. 1974. Viral disease of goslings. IV. Characteris-
      ation of the causal agent in tissue culture system. Acta Vet.Acad.
      Sci.Hung., 24, 287-292.
Kisary, J., Derzsy, D. and Horvàth, E. 1975. Az un.libainfluenza elleni

      szikimmunitàs jàrvànytani jelentösége. Magy.Ao.Lapja, <u>30</u>, 721-723.

Kisary, J. 1977. Immunological aspects of Derzsy's disease in goslings.
Avian Pathol., <u>6</u>, 327-334.

Kisary, J., Derzsy, D. and Mészàros, J. 1978. Attenuation of the goose parvovirus strain B. Laboratory and field trials of the attenuated mu-
tant for vaccination against Derzsy's disease. Avian Pathol., <u>7</u>,
397-406.

Kisary, J. 1979. Interaction in replication between the goose parvovirus
strain B and duck plague herpesvirus. Archives of Virol., <u>59</u>, 81-88.

Schettler, C.H. 1971a. Isolation of a highly pathogenic virus from geese
with hepatitis. Avian Dis., <u>15</u>, 323-325.

Schettler, C.H. 1971b. Virus hepatitis of geese. II. Host range of goose
hepatitis virus. Avian Dis., <u>15</u>, 809-823.

Schettler, C.H. 1979. Large scale investigation on the serological response
of breeder geese and Muscovy ducks to different types of live attenuated and inactivated goose hepatitis virus strain GHV-SHM 319.
Proc.Int.Conf. on Breeding and Geese Production, 197-202.